PENGUIN BOOKS

Middle-Age Spread Diet

Carolyn Gibson, author of eight best-selling diet and cook-books, is a recognised expert in weight management, stress and behavioural change. She has a double major degree in Psychology and Education and established her successful weight-loss groups in 1984.

Carolyn's motivational presentations make her a popular speaker at conferences, and she regularly appears on television as a celebrity chef. Carolyn is married with one daughter, Victoria, who is a qualified Personal Trainer; together they have co-authored several books.

Acknowledgements

Victoria Gibson-Clarke, Jac Holt, Gill Richmond.
Illustrations by Christine Brown.

Dedication

I dedicate this book to my mother, Lorna Wright, who weaves together my fragmented threads of thought and without her endless help my book would remain simply a collection of unconnected words.

Medical

It is advisable before starting any weight-loss plan to consult your family doctor. All care has been taken in compiling the exercise programme, but it is most important that all guidelines and instructions are carefully read and strictly adhered to. If you have any special health problems seek medical advice before continuing on the diet.

The recipes in this book have been created by the author. Any similarities to existing recipes are purely coincidental.

Middle-Age Spread Diet

Carolyn Gibson

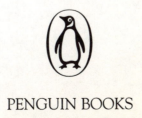

PENGUIN BOOKS

PENGUIN BOOKS

Published by the Penguin Group

Penguin Books (NZ) Ltd, cnr Airborne and Rosedale Roads, Albany,
Auckland 1310, New Zealand

Penguin Books Ltd, 80 Strand, London, WC2R 0RL, England

Penguin Group (USA) Inc., 375 Hudson Street, New York, NY 10014, United States

Penguin Books Australia Ltd, 250 Camberwell Road, Camberwell,
Victoria 3124, Australia

Penguin Books Canada Ltd, 10 Alcorn Avenue, Toronto,
Ontario, Canada M4V 3B2

Penguin Books (South Africa) (Pty) Ltd, 24 Sturdee Avenue, Rosebank,
Johannesburg 2196, South Africa

Penguin Books India (P) Ltd, 11, Community Centre, Panchsheel Park,
New Delhi 110 017, India

Penguin Books Ltd, Registered Offices: 80 Strand, London, WC2R 0RL, England

First published by Penguin Books (NZ) Ltd, 2003

1 3 5 7 9 10 8 6 4 2

Copyright © text Carolyn Gibson, 2003
Copyright © photographs Carolyn Gibson and Penguin Books, 2003

The right of Carolyn Gibson to be identified as the author of this work in terms of
section 96 of the Copyright Act 1994 is hereby asserted.

Designed by Mary Egan
Typeset by Egan-Reid Ltd
Printed in Australia by McPherson's Printing Group

ISBN 0 14 301876 0
A catalogue record for this book is available
from the National Library of New Zealand.

www.penguin.co.nz

Contents

Introduction

Middle-age spread gives new meaning to the term 'gone to pot!'

What a shock.

Our figures, once curvaceous in all the right places, now appear corrugated in all the wrong places, with a couple of rolls cascading down from our breasts to our stomachs.

A pot stomach – that is a new development. In the past our 'floating' additional kilos attached themselves to our hips and thighs. Now they accumulate around our middle. So what's going on? Prepare yourself because times are a changing.

From the age of 35 on our bodies undergo progressive age-related changes. Weight that in the past we may have been able to drop in a few days, or a week at the most, simply won't budge – or so it seems. Even women who have successfully managed their weight all their lives now find it difficult to maintain their weight even though their food intake is the same as before. After years of being slim they arrive in my classes unpleasantly surprised at what appears to be an overnight expansion of fat on their stomach.

I blamed menopause for my developing little pot.

After 23 years of maintaining my 28-kilo loss, it was a shock for me to discover small gains were depositing themselves around my waist and midriff. I'd heard the phrase 'my waist is thickening' – now I knew what it meant. I was horrified at the ability of my fat cells to remain fat and to resist all my efforts to regain my previous shape. I mean to say, I WRITE THE DIET BOOKS AND RUN THE CLASSES!

How could this happen to ME?

It became evident that what had worked for me, and others, in the past had to be re-evaluated. I needed to do some research.

When looking for an answer there is nothing more effective than experiencing the problem first-hand. Handing out advice is easy, but in order to be able to give good advice you must have 'been there, done that'. I have been teaching my weight-loss classes for 20 years, and while I had sympathised with older women about their abdominal fat I was at times sceptical about how hard they were actually trying. Now that I have joined their ranks I can understand their dilemma and frustration.

I became a subject in my own experiment of change. Over the past 18 months I have spent hours in the Medical School Library reading medical journals and examining the latest findings. I attended seminars, and pieced together my own experiences along with current research, which led me to make some major mind shifts from my previously held beliefs and practices. The first being my devotion to the humble potato, and meat and three vegetables at dinner. The second shift I had to make was to overcome my reluctance to exercise, which I flippantly dismissed on the grounds that I would never be taking my clothes off in public!

As a consequence I made changes to my own food intake and exercise routine while monitoring my results daily. I extended this to a trial group of women in my classes and compared their results against a control group. I identified the causes and I identified the changes that needed to be made. Out of this came the Middle-Age Spread Diet.

So what changes are needed?

Change is my constant theme and focus in this book.

We will discuss how we need to change our pattern of eating, increase our physical activity level, change our attitude and adjust our lifestyle. Most of us hate and avoid change, and although we may know the reasons why we are gaining weight, we don't confront them or deal with them. We say, 'I know the problem and I also know what I need to do.'

Well, if we know, why aren't we doing it? Sometimes the solution to a problem is right in front of our eyes and it isn't that we can't see it – we choose not to see it.

Why?

Because if we admit we know the answer it might mean we would have to take some action and that might mean we had to make some changes.

It all comes down to your motivation to succeed

What terminology are you using when you talk about losing weight?

Do you say 'I HAVE to lose weight'

or

do you say 'I WANT to lose weight'?

What's the difference?

Humour me here for a moment. I want you to say these sentences and experience the emotion attached to each one.

I HAVE to lose weight   =   bucket of cold water, compulsion, a chore, deprivation

I WANT to lose weight   =   motivation, excitement, desire for change

There is a difference. Feel it?

Success can balance on one simple word by creating a positive or a negative mindset. I am going to come back to your response in my conclusion. Keep an open mind and be receptive to change as we continue through the steps you will follow to begin the Middle-Age Spread Diet.

In Chapter 1 we will discuss how our middle-age spread is caused by a series of age-related chain reactions and we will examine these one by one.

Following this we will establish your Calorie Expenditure Rating, which will determine your daily food intake.

After that you'll find the section you've been waiting for –

The Middle-Age Spread Diet.

I have presented the diet in three stages.

We begin with the list of Daily Food Allowances. From these I have put together a meal-by-meal selection to lead you through the **timing** of the **seven daily intakes**. This is a training section to show you how you can use your Daily Food Allowances to your full advantage.

Finally, for those of you who prefer to follow a structured plan I have written four weeks of delicious meals, using recipes from the book. They will guide you through until you are ready to create your own menus.

Throughout the book I encourage you to visit me at my website www.carolyngibson.com for extra assistance, and you will find these pages marked with a 'Log In' icon.

It is all very well losing weight but maintenance is when many people lose the plot. I have written a practical, common-sense maintenance section for you to follow once you've reached your goal.

Exercise – well there had to be some and if I can do it, so can you. There are photographs and step-by-step instructions to show you exactly what to do.

Recipes are always popular and I have included a collection of some of my favourites. My current recipes reflect the trends towards foods of other cultures and café meals. They use lots of zesty lemon and spices, which activate not only the taste-buds but also our metabolic rate. Some treats await you there.

We can only make changes if we really **WANT** to **CHANGE**.

I made those changes and successfully controlled my middle-age spread.

You can too.

Let me tell you a little story

As a child I played the piano but stopped once I became a teenager. Over the years I never had the inclination or opportunity to play, but my memories of how well I had performed became colourful and somewhat enhanced.

This year, in a moment of madness, I saved a lovely hundred-year-old piano from going to the tip. Filled with excitement and enthusiasm I installed my borer-ridden piano in the garage with the thought that YES, I will play again! Off I went to lessons.

My piano teacher, Janet, welcomed me with a selection of pieces based on my claimed level of accomplishment. Within minutes we discovered my total inability to play anything. Confused fingers asking for direction did nothing for my rhythm.

'Have you thought about the timing, Carolyn?' Janet gently asked. Even that was a challenge. Have you tried counting, reading two lines at once and moving the fingers all at the same time? Recently I mean. In middle-age?

We dropped back to one hand, one line pieces in simple tempo, no sharps or flats. Deflated, every fibre of my body cried 'GIVE UP, what does it matter, who cares, I don't really have time for this – shoot the piano, send it to the tip!' After three weeks I began fabricating excuses why I couldn't continue my lessons, believing I was too old to start again. Accepting defeat is easy – and tempting.

But I didn't give up and I thank Janet's endless patience for that. I am now playing the piano, and it gives me lots of pleasure. I will never be amazing, but I practise when I can and I am making small and steady progress.

You might be wondering what has this got to do with middle-age spread?

Plenty.

Consider the similarities.

We start off with initial enthusiasm, which soon wears off when we aren't as good as we thought we were and success isn't immediate.

Timing is everything, and you will learn how important this is to the success of the Middle-Age Spread Diet. Establishing a rhythm of eating means you will eat regularly and not put yourself at risk of being hungry.

Too old to start again? You have a second chance – take it. Our past successes or failures have no bearing on what we can do right now. Don't accept defeat without even trying. Be happy to accept that small steady weight losses are better than small steady gains. It is easy for us to accept our weight gain as inevitable. Why even bother? What difference is it going to make?

Well, I believe it makes quite a big difference.

This is a book about my change of life and yours.

Chapter 1

Times are a Changing

Our Biological Clock

Have you ever lain in bed, late at night, and just listened to the clock tick?

Tick . . . tick . . . tick . . ., slow, steady and reliable. Our biological clock is also 'ticking'.

It has rung all the changes in our lives from birth to puberty, keeping to a 28-day cycle through to pregnancy and now menopause. When the pre-set alarm rings at middle-age it is a wake-up call to a series of collective events leading to 'the change of life'.

Did you ever stop to consider that the term 'change of life' is exactly that?

A change of life.

Take it literally – see it as an opportunity to change the direction of your life. We have let 'the change' become negatively associated solely with menopause and view the changes that occur in our bodies as an inevitable consequence.

Middle-age spread is not connected to the one single event of menopause but to a series of causal factors that are activated like a domino effect. Push one domino and the other dominoes fall in progression.

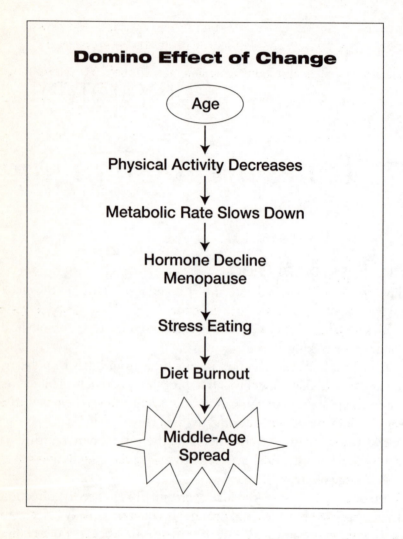

Domino Effect of Change

Age

↓

Physical Activity Decreases

↓

Metabolic Rate Slows Down

↓

Hormone Decline
Menopause

↓

Stress Eating

↓

Diet Burnout

↓

Middle-Age
Spread

What is the cause of middle-age spread?
The initial answer is simple –
AGE.

But age alone is not the culprit.

As we **age** there is a tendency to take things easy and **slow down,** which means our exercise and **physical activity levels decrease.**

This means we **lose lean body mass** and our **metabolic rate slows down.**

Hormones and neurotransmitters **decline** and our clock activates menopause,
which means we **re-distribute our excess fat,** suffer hot flushes, memory loss, panic attacks and mood swings.

This means we get **stressed,**
which means we **overeat,**
which means we try to **diet,**
which means we suffer **diet burnout,**
which means

WE GET FAT.

It also means that at middle-age we not only experience a weight gain, but also a change of shape and a change of risk.

Change of Shape
It is no wonder that the focus is placed on menopause when we find ourselves biologically defined as being either:
- Pre-menopausal – periods still regular
- Perimenopausal – time between having regular periods and no periods at all, or
- Postmenopausal – no period for one year

The emphasis is on the change in our menstrual cycle, but what is also changing is the location of where our body stores excess fat.

When we were **pre-menopausal** and in our reproductive years, fat was stored predominantly around our hips, thighs and buttocks, creating a pear-shaped body. The location of this storage was a biological function to ensure we could sustain life during pregnancy and breast-feeding.

When we are **perimenopausal** fat storage is distributed around our waist and abdomen region creating an apple-shaped body. Middle-age compounds an existing weight problem. Fat already stored on the hips and thighs does not magically up tents and move north to the abdomen. Rather we add to our problem by now storing new fat directly on the mid-region. Trousers that once sported belts are now traded for elastic-topped pants. Jeans, which in the past fitted with ease, now need to be zipped up as we lie flat on the bed. When we peel them off, the zip teeth leave a row of 'stitch' marks, making it look like we have just undergone open-stomach surgery!

You will be pleased to know that **postmenopausal** status brings us to a plateau in our lives where the age-related changes we have been experiencing tend to stabilise.

Change of Risk

The old saying that an apple a day keeps the doctor away is not applicable when it comes to the change in our body shape.

It is where the fat is distributed to that becomes of critical importance to our health.

In middle-age the focus changes from how overweight we are to where our fat is located. This change of shape caused by increased abdominal fat places us in the risk category for cardiovascular disease, late onset of non-insulin diabetes, hypertension and some forms of cancer. While abdominal fat stored on top of the abdominal muscle is of major concern, it is the excess visceral fat stored around the internal organs (e.g. liver, kidneys) that is considered to cause the greatest increase in health risks as fat may be released into the blood stream. Visceral fat, unlike abdominal fat, is not visible to the eye and can only be detected through computerised tomography (CT) scans. Unfortunately, its invisibility does not lessen its potential risk.

Change of Pace
Decreased physical activity

Clocks need to be wound up to keep them ticking or they will slow down and stop. As we age our bodies also need to be wound up and kept ticking if we are to avoid slowing down both physically and metabolically.

Age leads to decreased physical activity, resulting in loss of lean body mass (muscle), which is acknowledged to be the main determinant of middle-age spread.

Until recently I doubt that many women would have been familiar with the words **lean body mass**. Going to the gym to build up the muscles was for men, and walking was what we did to get us to the bus stop. How I managed those hills in my stiletto heels is still a mystery to me, never mind stepping onto the bus! But at least I walked a good distance every day. Ironically, as ill informed as we might have been, our muscles were probably in better shape. Modern technology and the car haven't been kind to our muscles, which don't get the daily workout doing the household chores that they once might have done.

I remember referring to 'sagging' as loss of skin tone – certainly not muscle loss. I mean, that is what sleeves are for – to cover it all up. However, as my daughter likes to point out to me, underneath my skin, somewhere, are muscles screaming out to be used. At an outdoor function I had pointed to a middle-aged woman who was wearing a sleeveless tank top and sporting extremely well-toned upper arms. 'Why aren't my arms like that?' I asked jealously. To which my daughter replied, 'Those arms, Mother, are serious arms – she lifts weights and exercises her muscles REGULARLY.' I was sorry I had asked!

Maybe the fact that we, as women, don't usually acknowledge that we have muscles is the reason we may not initially be concerned that we are losing them. But the state of our lean body mass is of vital importance to our ability to lose our middle-age spread.

Our lean body mass is metabolically active. This means it burns more calories than our fat cells, which are relatively inactive.

A shift from muscle to fat:
- makes it easier to gain weight
- makes it harder to maintain normal weight
- and increases our health risks.

But take heart, the problem is neither inevitable nor irreversible.

Studies show when our muscle and body fat remain stable there is also no metabolic decline with age.

A cross-observational study of postmenopausal women found that those who were physically active had less body and abdominal fat, which suggests that increased fitness is a useful tool in preventing unwanted age-related changes in body composition.

A study at Washington University found that middle-aged women who didn't exercise carried 38% of their weight as body fat compared with 25% in fit middle-aged women.

It has been reported that from the age of 35 onward, women who lead a sedentary lifestyle lose approximately 3.2 kilos of muscle every decade, and at the end of that time burn around 340 **fewer** calories per day. Think about it – the more muscle we lose the fewer calories our body burns and, if we continue to consume the same intake, the more calories we will have left over. These are then despatched to our fat cells for storage.

The point we need to understand here is . . .

**decreased physical activity is directly linked to the loss
of lean body mass,**

which contributes to the next causal factor,

the slowing down of our metabolic rate.

Metabolic Go Slow

We use, misuse, blame and totally misunderstand our metabolic rate – when it suits us.

So what is the metabolic rate?

The metabolic rate determines the number of calories we need to consume each day so that our energy intake equals our energy output.

To people who are slim we attribute a fast metabolic rate that, in our minds, immediately explains why they aren't overweight and why we are. It is always useful to be able to remove the blame away from ourselves – it couldn't possibly be anything to do with the food we ate or the alcohol we drank. Oh no – it's not us. Let's attribute the responsibility elsewhere. 'If it weren't for my metabolic rate, I wouldn't have this problem!'

Let me tell you that in clinical studies researchers have found that the majority of people tested who were convinced they suffered from a low metabolic rate were actually classified normal. So that shoots that theory down. It is also known that the bigger we are the higher our metabolic rate. This is because a larger body requires more energy to function.

What is not clearly understood is that as a consequence of age the metabolic rate changes, slows down, and we need fewer calories.

Metabolic Go Slow doesn't occur overnight. The body has been gently putting the brakes on since we turned 20 years of age.

From 20 up to 50 years, our metabolic rate is decreasing at a rate of between 2% to 5% every decade, with an average of 4%. Between 50 and 60 years, we are less physically active and the metabolic rate decreases by 10%.

Let's look at how this Metabolic Go Slow compounds to cause a gradual, but steady, increase in our weight.

Age	Approx. decrease	Cumulative decrease
20 to 30 years	4% decrease	4% requires 60 calories reduction per day
30 to 40 years	4% decrease	8% requires 120 calories reduction per day
40 to 50 years	4% decrease	12% requires 180 calories reduction per day
50 to 60 years	10% decrease	22% requires 340 calories reduction per day

So between the ages of 20 and 60 years our metabolic rate decreases a total of 22%, and after 60 we need 340 calories less each day just to maintain our existing weight.

Researchers have found that, on average, women between the ages of 35 and 55 years gain approximately 500 grams per year. This doesn't sound much, but in those 20 years it can result in a total gain of 10 kilos or more. Some studies reported gains of 4.5 kilos in just 3 years. Note that these are average gains and I warn you that 10 kilos is a moderate gain for those who do not take action. Gaining as little as 125 grams a week adds up to 6.5 kilos a year.

What is important to understand here is that this is what happens even though we are not eating more food. As our metabolic rate slows down we are gaining weight on the same intake we were able to maintain on in the past.

The solution to the Metabolic Go Slow requires a two pronged attack.

1. Increase physical activity

I am going to be repetitive here to emphasise the point that it is the loss of lean body mass, due to the decrease in physical activity, due to age, that is the major cause of our metabolic slow down. It is an increase in physical activity that will increase our lean body mass and, in turn, increase our metabolic rate.

To lift our metabolic rate we need to reduce body fat and increase muscle.

To do this we are going to EXERCISE and the best form of exercise for us is weight bearing. Now this doesn't mean that you will be built like a Russian shot-put competitor, so don't panic that you are going to end up muscle bound. I encourage you to join me in a workout plan specially created for us (page 129) which will strengthen and tone our bodies.

Remember, if we WANT a change, we must make a change.

2. Decrease your calorie intake

The Middle-Age Spread Diet provides all the guidelines you need.

When decreasing your calorie intake it is important that you do not dramatically cut back below 1200 calories per day. To do so would make the fat cells fight back and cause your metabolic rate to drop by up to 15%, which would make it a self-defeating strategy.

Unfortunately, our bodies cannot tell the difference between a food reduction, intentionally caused by ourselves, or by a real scarcity of food, such as in the case of famine. A sudden excessive shortfall in our calorie intake causes the body to go into survival mode, where it lowers the metabolic rate to conserve energy while it assesses whether the reduction in intake is temporary or long term.

So, strange as it seems, too low an intake slows your metabolic rate and makes it more difficult for you to lose weight. On the other hand eating creates what is called dietary thermogenesis, or Thermic Effect. In fact, after eating a meal our metabolic rate increases by between 10% and 35% and remains stimulated for a period of 2 to 3 hours afterwards. With this Thermic Effect we can burn 25 calories per meal which is great news for those of us who love to eat.

Food itself is not the enemy – the enemy is over-consumption.

Make a Change

Can we reactivate our metabolic rate?
ABSOLUTELY

Apply the 3 E formula for Metabolic Speed-Up

Exercise – increases lean body mass, which
increases the metabolic rate (refer page 129)
+
Eat regular, small meals every day as explained
in the Middle-Age Spread Diet (refer page 45).
Do not cut back below the food
allowances in List A
+
Establish your Resting Metabolic Rate (RMR)
and recheck it regularly as your weight
and fitness levels change (refer page 41)

E + E + E = Metabolic Speed-Up

The slowing metabolic rate is one link in the chain, but when the hormones also start declining, batten down the hatches, **menopausal woman on the loose.**

Hormones on the Rampage

BEWARE – I am a menopausal woman and I have a gun – which would make me dangerous if I could only remember who I am and what these keys are for!

Memory loss, mood swings, unpredictability –

We are inclined to blame our hormones for everything that happens to us. 'It isn't my fault it's my hormones.' I read an interesting article that stated when something goes wrong for a woman it is blamed on her internal situation (time of the month, hormones, menopause).

When something goes wrong for a man it is blamed on something external to him – the traffic, the job, the dog, not him.

I never had a sweet tooth until I became menopausal. I started off just looking for a little boost, until one day it turned into a jellybean tidal wave. It reached a point where I had to ration out my jellybeans into bags and seal up my daily supply. I was like an addict who couldn't be trusted with the whole bag at once. The craving was intense and I became a secret sugarholic.

Now I wanted to know why.

I discovered the answer in research findings that attributed sweet cravings to the decrease in estrogen, serotonin and endorphin levels.

Declining hormone levels – well that made some sense. At last I had somewhere to place the blame. And I laid it squarely on the fact that I was menopausal. I heard myself loudly claiming, 'I am being hormonally challenged! I can't remember everything – I am menopausal.' On and on I went. What a wonderful excuse for everything that happened – nothing was ever going to be my fault again.

But can we hold menopause responsible for our middle-age spread? NO.

Middle-age spread is not a consequence of menopause – menopause is a consequence of age.

Position menopause where it should be – a point of change on our transitional biological time-line. It is the decrease in estrogen and our neurotransmitters that are of interest here, not menopause itself.

From around the age of 35 on (or during menopause), estrogen production goes into decline. This is when our fat cells are on our side. They detect the drop in estrogen and begin to assist in the production of estrogen for us. As the ovaries stop production the fat cells begin. Within this theory it is proposed that the fat cells around the waist increase in size as abdominal fat is located more conveniently to the liver, which produces the enzymes required to produce estrogen from testosterone. Although we may be reluctant to acknowledge the presence of male hormones in our body we do have testosterone, which is also in a state of decline, and this in turn contributes to the loss of our lean body mass.

The only blame we can attribute to our hormones is that the decrease in estrogen contributes to the redistribution of excess fat to the abdomen. Our hormones don't create the excess fat – we do. It is far more likely that our choice of food, alcohol and lack of exercise are the causal factors. In fact, studies have found a high correlation between the level of alcohol consumed and weight gained after menopause.

So don't hit the bottle and blame the hormones.

An area of decline that is overshadowed by all the headlines directed at estrogen deficiency is the decrease in two important neurotransmitters, serotonin and endorphins. Neurotransmitters are brain chemicals that send messages from one neuron (brain cell) to another, and they are extremely influential in many aspects of our lives.

Serotonin is our stabilizer, it calms us down, makes us feel good, and satisfies our cravings. There are no prizes for guessing what stimulates the increase of this chemical from the brain.

Yes, it's CARBOHYDRATES AND SUGARS.

I have lost count of the number of times women have told me that their problem food is BREAD.

Lack of serotonin leads to food cravings (developing a sweet tooth – jellybeans!), sleep deprivation, mood swings and memory loss.

Do you remember that when we experienced PMT we had sugar cravings? This was due to a reduction in our estrogen level before menstruation. The same cravings kick in now, but this time they are due more to the reduction in our serotonin level.

If our serotonin level is low we begin to crave food that will give it a boost. Carrot sticks just don't do the job! When women tell me they keep carrot sticks in the fridge 'for emergencies', I ask, 'Do you enjoy eating them?' Invariably the answer is a shocked 'No!'

When we need a particular food and we don't satisfy that urge, it doesn't go away. We could eat a whole sack of carrots and still want a slice of bread. We are far better off having the slice of bread with butter and jam that will satisfy the craving by the release of serotonin and endorphins, and allow us to move on.

While we are on the topic of sugars, I feel it is important to briefly discuss the sugar versus artificial sweetener debate. When you crave something sweet, do not under any circumstances try to satisfy the urge with an artificially sweetened product. If your body needs sugar give it sugar. Don't try to trick the body. The taste-buds on the tongue only acknowledge whether the foods are sweet, sour, bitter or salty. As an artificial sweetener passes across the tongue a signal is sent to the brain that 'sweet' is on the way in. But no genuine 'sweet' is processed and the release of serotonin is not activated. If you weren't craving sugars before – you are now.

Artificial sweeteners do not satisfy sugar cravings or replace low blood sugars.

We didn't gain weight because we didn't eat diet products. We don't need to eat them to lose weight. Dump all your diet products and feel the joy of opening up the cupboards and fridge to normal, everyday foods that will be more satisfying, nutritious and healthy.

This doesn't mean you can binge on sugar. Getting a quick fix from sugar is only short-lived. The boost is followed by blood sugar levels plummeting. Sugar fixes only last for 20 to 30 minutes and then we need another hit. When carbohydrate and fat are combined the satisfaction lasts longer, which is one of the reasons I will be encouraging you to eat your toast with butter and jam in the late afternoon.

What about the endorphins?

I am sure you have heard people talking about experiencing an 'athlete's high'. When our endorphins are low we feel stressed, feel pain, can't think clearly and our energy levels are depleted. Endorphins, our natural uppers, are activated not only with exercise but also by the foods we eat, fats being one of them. It is no wonder some people suffer depression when they follow an exceptionally low-fat diet.

HRT

We can't move on from hormones without briefly touching on Hormone Replacement Therapy. HRT – Hormone Replacement Therapy, the name says it all really. We are trying to replace a hormone that is in a natural state of decline. I want to stress the words **natural state of decline**. Menopause is not a disease but a natural transition no different from the puberty we passed through and survived. Therapy? I find this an interesting word in association with this problem and wonder whether it is our hormones that need therapy or us.

A vet once told me that he doesn't treat the animals, he treats the pets' owners.

HRT and weight gain

Medical researchers argue that weight gain does not occur as a result of taking HRT but rather blame it on other age factors. I differ on this point of view and have found that many women on HRT experience a gain of between 6 and 10 kilos. I acknowledge that I am making this assessment on a sample of women (a large sample) who attend my weight-loss classes – so my opinion could be viewed as biased and my results invalid. However, my involvement with women over the past 20 years has given me access to thousands of women and their histories and I have always found that women's shared experiences provide a remarkably accurate assessment.

I have always been personally opposed to the use of HRT, and I made the choice to go through the transition of menopause without the assistance of any drugs or herbal remedies. In the light of recent medical evidence I believe my decision not to use HRT has been proved to be the correct one for me. However, I do accept that for some women HRT has been beneficial and improved the quality of their lives.

Whether to take HRT is not a decision to be made here. Broaden your knowledge of the subject, discuss it with a trusted medical practitioner and follow your own female intuition.

Make a Change

1. Select foods that contain phytoestrogens, are fresh and nutrient dense (refer page 116).

2. DO NOT, under any circumstances, use artificial sweeteners. If you need sugar – use sugar.

3. Avoid processed foods and foods wrapped in plastic film.

4. Discuss the pros and cons of HRT with your doctor.

5. Change your attitude to menopause. It is not a disease; we all go through it and it will pass eventually. With a bit of luck we won't even remember!

With all the physical and psychological changes we experience at this stage of our lives it is no wonder we end up feeling stressed, and we know what stress leads to – STRESS EATING.

Stress Eating

Must do lunch!

Recently I bumped into an old school friend. A brief chat finished with promises of 'must do lunch'. I commented that this wasn't how we had perceived our lives would be in our fifties. We thought it would be lunches with the girls, tennis, grandchildren visiting, patchwork and leisure. The reality is that most of the women I know have never worked so hard or been under such stress as they are now.

Some are working full-time, others are minding their grandchildren to help their children who have returned to the work-force. Few have time to call their own and it is all taking its toll. It sometimes feels as if we are holding a handful of different balloons, or tasks, just managing to keep a tight grip on them all, and another balloon is thrust into our hands. The scramble to balance and add in this new balloon causes us to momentarily let a few escape. Our attempt to regather them becomes a moment of losing the plot, which leads to our stress being intensified. Lack of control over the situation and no outlet for the sense of helplessness are two of the biggest causes of chronic stress.

Many of us do not recognise the stress we are under; we just plod on, honouring our commitments, giving very little attention to our own needs, and OVER-EATING.

I want to ask you a question.

Do you eat when you are under stress?

When I asked this question in my classes, 95% responded with 'Yes!'

The next question is more important to our understanding of stress eating. Do you eat while the actual stress is occurring, or after the event? It may surprise you to learn that most of us eat afterwards, not at the height of the stressful situation.

It is unlikely that many of us have ever wondered why we do this. The explanation goes way back to the days when we were the hunters and the hunted. Our bodies are wired for stress, and still react to danger in the same way as they did in prehistoric times – by activating a survival mechanism to keep us safe in the wild. These days we may not be at risk from wild beasts but our modern world holds its own dangers. Encountering an aggressive dog, a sudden noise as we open the car door, experiencing a burglary, family conflict, financial burdens or having your bag snatched (which happened to me overseas on the way to catch a flight) all result in STRESS!

What we experience in these situations is a rush of adrenaline (a hormone released from the adrenal glands into the blood stream), which activates the fight-or-flight response. This prepares us for emergency conditions and a series of responses are activated – fast.

Stored energy is released from our muscles, our heart rate increases, our breathing becomes shallow and rapid, and clarity of the brain is heightened, while both the immune system and HUNGER are **suppressed**. All attention is focused on the real or perceived threat. Usually the threat is a false alarm or a minor emergency and does not require drastic action. We certainly aren't in a state of fight or flight.

If the stress had required physical action the hormones would have been used to give our muscles strength to fight the danger. Now we have all the unused released adrenaline circulating in our blood stream and we don't need it. And that is the problem.

The energy (fat) released is now returned to the fat cells. You will remember that during the stressful event hunger was suppressed, or turned off. In the recovery mode our bodies are seeking to replace the lost energy source and it is NOW that we begin our stress eating.

Our body thinks we have been fighting the wild beast and believes it is necessary to replace the energy released. So we feel hungry. Too often we believe this overwhelming desire to eat/binge is a weakness on our part and emotionally based. It is important that you understand the need is primarily physical and strong. You haven't given in, you have responded to a biological function.

Now that you know the reason for your hunger you will know how to deal with it. If you really have been fighting or fleeing you are allowed to eat – need to eat – so give the body what it needs. If the event was a false alarm your best response is to imitate the 'flight' part and instead of eating take a long walk to use up the energy.

On the other hand, the people who find they can't eat after experiencing stress are those whose stress hormones are continually triggered. They are in a state of constant turmoil or anxiety and hunger is turned off. While this might seem to be the ideal state, this level of stress is most detrimental to our health, because when the hunger button is turned off, so too is our immune button. There are many studies that link some forms of cancer to high stress levels.

When our bodies are in a constant state of stress, high levels of insulin and cortisol discourage fat being used, and encourage our fat cells to store fat in close proximity to the liver and adrenal glands for quick access ready for the next emergency. Fat storage around the waist is increased just where you don't want it.

So remember next time stress strikes – WALK.

Continual stress leads to burnout and we will discuss that next.

Diet Burnout

Age is a factor in a condition I call Diet Burnout. If you are 35 years or older you have probably been on ten or more diets during your life, lost countless kilos, and gained twice the amount back. You can claim to have tried every diet on the market and consider yourself a professional with enough expertise to appear as a contestant on Master Mind, your specialist subject DIETS.

Yes, you are most definitely a candidate for Diet Burnout. Check out these symptoms:

Emotional exhaustion	–	insomnia, finding it difficult to make simple decisions, feeling overwhelmed by day-to-day chores
Depersonalisation	–	no sense of humour, cynicism, short fuse
Feelings of low personal accomplishment	–	frustration, helplessness, not producing results, and finally GIVING UP.

Sound familiar? We keep trying but keep hitting the wall and it has a negative effect on our feelings of self-esteem and in our belief that we can achieve our goal. Don't underestimate the effects of burnout, you don't have to be an executive to experience it. Burnout can be extremely detrimental to our wellbeing.

There are two key issues in relation to weight loss – one psychological and one physical.

Firstly, we experience a lack of motivation due to years of continually pushing the I AM ON A DIET button. How many times can we crank up our enthusiasm for losing weight and feel the apprehension of telling our family and friends we are starting yet another diet? We begin to worry about a repeat of our previous regains. We fear failing yet again. At this stage of our lives our decision to lose weight is usually based on panic because of an approaching event or a health scare, and so we bite the bullet, do what is necessary in the short-term, but make no long-term behavioural changes. We usually succeed for the event or checkup, but then we return to our old eating habits and back comes the weight.

What a surprise! What a disappointment!

Secondly, there is a physical effect from our years of dieting. There are repercussions from the constant losses and recurring weight gains. Each time we lose weight and regain it we are changing our body composition. Weight loss is made up not only of fat but also muscle and water. Let me give you an example.

Lose 20 kilos			Regain lost 20 kilos		
Fat	=	10 kilos	Fat	=	15 kilos
Muscle	=	5 kilos	Muscle	=	0
Water	=	5 kilos	Water	=	5 kilos

You can see that if you have continually repeated this process over the last 20 years it is now having a dramatic effect on your present efforts to lose weight.

Studies have found weight cycling significantly influenced fat storage on the abdominal region. So, in the example above you would have lost 10 kilos of fat from selected parts of your body, but on regaining 15 kilos of fat there is a high probability most of it will end up on your abdomen.

We are not dealing with the same body as we were in the beginning. Our body composition has changed and so too has the way we must approach weight loss. The old game plan isn't working anymore. So clear the field and begin to play by a new set of rules.

Make a Change

1. It won't get any easier to lose weight – do it now and get it right.

2. Exercise. Get up earlier in the mornings and go for a walk before breakfast. You will feel more invigorated if you get up the moment you wake up, or when the alarm rings. Resist snuggling back down – GET UP.

3. Create a routine with your eating – no big gaps. Use your fruit, carbohydrate and fat allowances to help keep your serotonin and endorphin levels high. We want a natural high.

4. Try to create a pocket of the day that is your 'switch-off time'. Have a bath with special relaxing oils – lock the door and read a magazine.

5. Incorporate foods rich in Vitamin C and other nutrients into your day.

6. Understand yourself – keep a record of what is happening to you on the Personal Analysis Sheet in the Appendix (refer page 242) or download your sheet from my website www.carolyngibson.com.

LOG IN
Personal analysis

Chapter 2

Do I have to get on the Scales?

'Don't tell me – I don't want to know.'

I have lost count of the number of times I have heard this statement from a client who did not want to be weighed or for the weight to be recorded on her card. Although I can appreciate that we want to remain in a state of denial about our weight and not confront reality, you do need to know where you are positioned before you can proceed. Let me assure you that later on you will want to know your starting weight, so that you can enjoy the satisfaction of what you have achieved. You don't want to be guessing that you 'think you have lost 3 kilos' – you will want to know. Without taking some form of measurement you can't assess whether what you are doing is giving you the result you deserve or desire.

The scales are not used to make a judgement on you personally. However, this is the impression I get when greeting women at my class. The simple question of 'how was your week' is almost invariably answered with 'I will tell you when I get on the scales!'

The important issue here is that having reached middle-age the scales do not necessarily tell us the whole story. They do not indicate the change in the distribution of our fat storage onto the abdomen and central region of our bodies. When it comes to our health, it isn't only a matter of what we weigh, but where we are storing the excess fat.

To establish whether your weight is placing your health at risk, we are going to do a risk assessment test. I have listed the steps for you to follow below.

STEP ONE

Establish Waist Circumference Measurement

Measure your waist at the smallest circumference. [   ] cm

If your waist measurement equals **88 cm (35 inches) or greater**, you are considered to be in the **high-risk** category and need to lose weight. If your waist measurement is **less than 88 cm** proceed to

⟶ **STEP TWO**

Establish Waist-to-Hip Ratio (WHR)

Fill in your waist and hip measurements in the boxes below

Waist Measurement = [   ] cm   (e.g. [100] cm)

Hip Measurement   = [   ] cm   (e.g. [110] cm)

Divide the waist measurement by the hip measurement.

(e.g. WHR = 100 **divided** by 110 = **0.91**)

For women, an answer of 0.8 or higher indicates an increased health risk and weight loss is required.

Having established your risk factor we will now establish your Body Mass Index.

Working out your Body Mass Index

The Body Mass Index (BMI) is a formula used to estimate the proportion of your body that consists of fat. It is currently considered the best guide for calculating a healthy weight range for people aged between 20 and sixty-five.

Let's look at the figures. We will work through this together as many of us are mathematically shy. If you would like assistance with any of these equations you can log onto my website and simply fill in your details on screen. The programme will give you your answer.

To work out the equation divide your weight in kilos by your height in metres squared.

$$\text{BMI} = \frac{\text{Weight in kilograms}}{\text{Height in metres}^2}$$

For example:

| Weight in kilos | $\dfrac{82}{1.65 \times 1.65}$ | = | $\dfrac{82}{3}$ | = | **BMI** | = | 27 |
| Height × height | | | | | | | |

| Your weight | $\dfrac{\Box}{\Box \times \Box}$ | = | $\dfrac{\Box}{\Box}$ | = | Your BMI | = | $\Box$ |
| Your height × height | | | | | | | |

The answer that you get with this equation is NOT your weight in kilos but it is the factor that we will use to establish your healthy weight range.

BMI Guideline

BMI under 20	You are underweight
20–24	Your weight is within the ideal range
25–27	You are slightly overweight
Over 27	You are overweight and at risk of weight-related problems

Set your Target Weight

Use the Weight Guidelines Table (refer page 36) to establish a realistic target weight. Note that there is a wide range, and I recommend that to begin with you position your weight in the upper half of your height–age range.

How Much Gain is Okay?

I view the body, prior to middle-age, like a well-maintained city, contained within a clearly defined boundary. Gradually, new housing moves to the city limits and then, what appears to be overnight, a sudden population explosion and the city spreads to the suburbs. You know how you drive past a field one day and it's a housing development the next.

So how do these boundaries move without us being aware of the changes? Easy, we kept moving the boundary pegs.

Have you ever leapt off the scales in horror, and said 'THAT'S IT! I might be 68 kilos today but I will never let myself go above that.' Then at the next weigh in you're 70.1. You do a quick convert back to old weight system to find you're just over 11 stone. 'I will NEVER let myself get to 11½ stone,' you say. NEVER? Oh dear – now it is 12 stone. And so it goes on – literally.

Saying 'I don't know how this has happened, I was quite slim yesterday' is living in a state of delusion. The weight did not occur overnight. It is the accumulation of small, unacknowledged gains that have slowly increased without us taking action.

Weight Guidelines Table

Based on Body Mass Index (BMI)

Age Group		35–44	45–54	55–64+

Your Height

Ft/Inches	Metres	Weight Kg	Weight Kg	Weight Kg
4ft 8 in	1.42	41–53	41–55	41–57
4ft 9 in	1.44	43–55	43–57	43–59
4ft 10 in	1.47	44–57	44–59	44–62
4ft 11 in	1.50	46–59	46–62	46–64
5ft 0 in	1.52	48–61	48–64	48–66
5ft 1 in	1.55	50–63	50–65	50–68
5ft 2 in	1.57	52–65	52–67	52–70
5ft 3 in	1.60	53–67	53–69	53–72
5ft 4 in	1.62	55–69	55–72	55–74
5ft 5 in	1.65	57–71	57–74	57–77
5ft 6 in	1.68	59–73	59–77	59–79
5ft 7 in	1.70	61–76	61–79	61–82
5ft 8 in	1.72	63–78	63–82	63–84
5ft 9 in	1.75	65–81	65–84	65–87
5ft 10 in	1.78	67–83	67–87	67–90
5ft 11 in	1.80	69–86	69–89	69–93
6ft 0 in	1.83	71–88	71–92	71–96

Source: 'Food for Health' Report of Nutrition Taskforce to the Department of Health, 1991.

When it comes to an acceptable weight gain it appears we are being lulled into a false sense of security. Research findings suggest that a weight gain of 4 to 5 kilos in midlife is acceptable. This is based on an assessed weight gain of between 500 grams to one kilo per year. DO YOU REALLY THINK YOU CAN ONLY GAIN 500 GRAMS A YEAR! Let's face it, a dinner out, a weekend away, Christmas – get on the scales and see how much you have gained and I am sure it will be more than 500 grams in just one week. And it doesn't get any better. It is estimated that women, who are already overweight when they reach midlife, can gain a further 10 kilos during perimenopause.

I believe we need to apply three simple rules, and the first is:

Don't get any bigger!

Even if you were only to hold the weight you are right now, you would still be ahead of what you could be in 5 years. Think of the slow gains of just 125 grams a week, which add up to 6.5 kilos (or just over one stone in the old language) per year.

If we take no positive action about our weight it will not stay the same. Of that you can be sure!

The second rule is:

Be realistic in your expectations.

A weekly average weight loss of 400 grams is perfect. In the old days, we thought it was ideal to lose one pound a week and the medical profession still do. We went metric and with it went all common sense. Now women want to lose one kilo a week (2lb 3oz). This is neither realistic nor sustainable.

Do you know that in order to lose one pound (450 grams) you need to eliminate 3500 calories out of your food plan for the week. I find it useful to explain this to women who don't value their 400 gram loss. When they tell me they put the effort in I can tell them honestly that I KNOW they did. Another useful piece of information is how a 400-grams-a-week loss adds up to a total of 20.8 kilos in year. Now that does have value!

There will be times when you have followed a perfect week and you don't lose weight.

Shock – horror! You begin to question what you have done 'wrong', self-doubt starts to creep in and you worry that the weight loss has stalled.

I want you to listen carefully to this and don't panic. Throughout your weight loss there will be periods of consolidation. Think of it like this. Let's say you have lost 6 kilos in 10 weeks. That is an excellent loss, but as far as your physiological body is concerned, there may be a problem. If you were living off the land, hunting and gathering, and you unexpectedly lost 6 kilos in a relatively short period of time, what could the implications be? A famine, war, loss of crops, injury and inability to hunt? We may have evolved from our primitive environment to 24-hour supermarkets, but we are still wired to respond to any threat to our survival. In the event of a short fall in energy intake, the body adjusts to the situation by holding its position until the safety of the situation has been assessed. Is the reduced energy intake constant?

Understand that this is what is happening and you will feel more confident. I can assure you that when you continue with the food plan, your weight will continue to go down. Every week in my classes I have some women who are disappointed because their loss for the week is only 200 or 300 grams. The following week they can't believe their loss has leapt to over 1 kilo. Don't concede defeat at the first hurdle.

Many women tell me 'I need to lose ALL this fat'. Understand one point right here. What we want to achieve is a loss of excess fat, and even a woman of average weight has approximately 30 to 50 billion, yes billion, fat cells. The body fat of a woman who is not overweight can weigh in the range of 15 to 18 kilos – we need these fat cells.

The third rule is:

Weigh yourself once a week only.

I don't want you leaping on and off the scales every day during the week. There is no surer way to drive yourself crazy and to send you off seeking solace at the fridge. Understand that there will be natural fluctuations in your weight through the week.

There is no justice in weight loss. The body allows the weight to be shed in its own pattern of time. We are conditioned to be rewarded within a particular time frame for the work done. You have put in seven good days and rightly expect a result. But it doesn't work like that. It is a bit like reporting to the wages clerk on a Friday for your pay to be told 'I know you worked hard all week, but I don't know when I'll pay you. I might pay you today, or maybe next Tuesday, but you will be paid.' We would never accept this in a work situation, but in relation to our weight loss, it is exactly how we must view it.

As I tell my clients – you might weigh with me every Wednesday, but your body doesn't know that this is the day it has to register the loss.

When will we be satisfied?

One night in my class, a woman who had lost 1.9 kilos in one week stated to the class that she was unhappy with this loss as she had expected to lose AT LEAST 2 kilos. Now let me point out that this was not her first week on the diet when we can achieve higher than average losses due to fluid loss. I felt my temperature gauge rising, and it was a shock to everyone when I rather loudly exclaimed, 'WHEN WILL WE EVER BE SATISFIED!'

My concern was twofold. If we can't be happy with a 1.9 kilo loss – what will we be happy with? Secondly, how would you have felt sitting in that class, pleased with your loss of 400 grams, only to hear that 1.9 kilos was not good enough? Every gram we lose is a huge achievement.

It never ceases to amaze me how we, as rational, intelligent women, lose all sense of objectivity when it comes to our weight. We take control and responsibility in other areas of our lives, quickly dealing with the problems thrown at us. Our weight gain problems can also be solved by applying the same level of application.

To resolve a problem we first need to identify it. Spend a few minutes NOW to list the reasons why you are not losing weight. Be honest!

6 reasons why I am not losing weight:

(e.g. I am skipping lunch.)

1.

2.

3.

4.

5.

6.

Acknowledge these reasons and deal with them.

Get the picture?

Some years ago a friend of mine who was overweight came to me in tears and asked for my help. Knowing her past history of not sticking to diets I made a deal: 'Let me take your photograph before you start so that we have a record to look back on.' With huge reluctance and a sense of desperation she agreed to the mug shot. 'NEVER show me that photo – NEVER!' Ten months later, when she had lost 22 kilos, curiosity got the better of her and she said 'show me the photo'. This time there were tears of joy.

Keep a record of your progress – just like my friend you will be pleased that you did.

LOG IN
Download Record
Card

As Simple as A B C

We are all individuals and our experience of ageing, menopause and energy expenditure will differ. Research has found that a calorie intake sufficient for a slightly overweight person is too low for someone who is heavier.

To allow us to personalise the programme to suit your individual requirements we have employed a method for assessing your calorie level based on a Resting Metabolic Rate (RMR) formula, which you will record on your Personal Profile (refer page 44) and use to establish your Calorie Expenditure Rating (CER) as either A B or C.

If you are a B or a C you will be allocated, in some food categories, either an extra serving or a slightly larger sized portion than an A will receive. Make your selection from the correct column according to your rating. Use the formula below to find your rating.

Calorie Expenditure Rating (CER)

We are going to work through this together.
First we will work out your Resting Metabolic Rate

1. Establish your weight in kilos. ☐

2. Multiply your weight by 22.

   | kgs | x | 22 | = RMR   = ☐

3. Select your Activity Level % from the chart below.
   Tick box
   ☐ **Light Activity**   **20% of RMR**
   ☐ **Moderate Activity**   **30% of RMR**
   ☐ **High Activity**   **40% of RMR**

4. Multiply your RMR by Activity Level %.

   | RMR | x | % | = Active Metabolic Rate (AMR)   = ☐

5. Add them together.

   | RMR | x | AMR | = Calorie Expenditure Rating (CER) = ☐

When it comes to maths, I always like to see an example.

Weight in kilos e.g. $\quad\quad$ = 82 kilos

Multiply by $\quad\quad\quad\quad$ × 22 $\quad\quad\quad$ = 1804

$\quad\quad\quad\quad\quad\quad\quad\quad\quad\quad\quad\quad$ = Resting Metabolic Rate (RMR)

Establish activity level e.g. moderate

Percentage for moderate is 30%

In your calculator multiply RMR 1804 × 0.3 $\quad$ = 541

$\quad\quad\quad\quad\quad\quad\quad\quad\quad\quad\quad\quad$ = Active Metabolic Rate (AMR)

Add RMR (1804) and AMR (541) $\quad\quad\quad$ = 2345

$\quad\quad\quad\quad\quad\quad\quad\quad\quad\quad\quad\quad$ = **Calorie Expenditure Rating (CER)**

In this example the answer is (2345). This would classify you as a C Rating (see below).

If your Calorie Expenditure Rating (CER) is:

• between 1600 and 1900	select from the A List
• between 1901 and 2300	select from the B List
• 2301 or over	select from the C List

Once a month reassess your Calorie Expenditure Rating as this will require adjustment due to changes in your weight.

Why the ABC Ratings?

Your resting Metabolic Rate (RMR) determines how much energy is needed to keep your body at rest. Think of it like your car. At its RMR your car is idling at the lights. When going full throttle up the hill your car uses more fuel. Like the car, when you are physically active you need more fuel (calories).

When establishing your Calorie Expenditure Rating (CER) an amount is added to your RMR to allow for your level of activity. When you select your Activity Level Percentage decide if you are speeding or just taking a leisurely drive.

Another point of comparison – a large car uses more petrol than a small car over the same distance. That is why, on the Middle-Age Spread Diet, we have formulated the A B C Ratings and have allocated larger servings for those who have the most weight to lose.

Now that wasn't too difficult was it? So don't be put off when you see the formula, you can work it out, but if you would like some help, you can visit my website and simply type in your data. Your Calorie Expenditure Rating will be worked out for you.

Why didn't I tell you that at the beginning? Well, I like to set you little challenges.

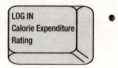

At last it is time for us to begin the Middle-Age Spread Diet!

MY PERSONAL PROFILE

Date   _____

Current Weight (kilos)   [   ]

Waist (cms)   [   ]

Height (metres)   [   ]

Hips (cms)   [   ]

Waist to Hip Ratio (WHR) refer page 33   [   ]

(WHR) = Waist divided by Hip

Body Mass Index (BMI) refer page 34   [   ]

(BMI) = (Weight) divided by (height squared)

Resting Metabolic Rate (RMR) refer page 41   [   ]

(RMR) = Weight multiplied by 22

Calorie Expenditure Rating (CER) refer page 41   [   ]

(CER) = RMR plus AMR

TARGET WEIGHT refer BMI Tables page 36   [   ]

Use this page to record your personal details.

It will be interesting to refer back to when you reach your
target weight.

Chapter 3

The Middle-Age Spread Diet

▶ Change the Timing

▶ Daily Food Allowances

▶ Meal by Meal – learning to put it together

▶ Food Planners – three weeks of planned meals to get you started

▶ On the Run – a planner for a busy week

Change the Timing
Timing is everything.

WHEN we eat is as important as **WHAT** we eat.

Once we reach middle-age **timing** and **distribution** are the key factors in successful weight reduction.

What worked for us in the past may not be effective now – it is time for **CHANGE.**

This change begins with allocating our food allowances into seven daily mini-meals eaten at specified time slots – applying the scallop effect to eating. This minimises the peaks and troughs of hunger and reduces the risk of over-eating later in the day.

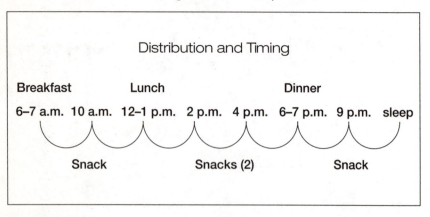

Distribution and Timing

Breakfast   Lunch   Dinner

6–7 a.m. 10 a.m. 12–1 p.m. 2 p.m. 4 p.m. 6–7 p.m. 9 p.m. sleep

Snack   Snacks (2)   Snack

By following the Middle-Age Spread Diet we are going to eat smaller, more frequent meals and set our timing to coincide with our metabolic rate, which is highest between 6.00 a.m. and 6.00 p.m., peaking between 11.00 a.m. and 2.00 p.m., when the sun is at its highest point.

This is the time we need to consume our largest intake of energy. In our busy lifestyles it is easy to fall into the trap of skipping breakfast, snacking at lunch, overeating in the afternoon, eating a large dinner and consuming our largest intake from 6.00 p.m. onwards. Bringing our food forward into the day allows us to process it more efficiently, while we are still active and the metabolic rate is functioning on high. Ideally we will consume 55% of our daily calorie intake before 2.00 p.m. We achieve this by not skipping breakfast, by eating a mid-morning snack, and by making lunch an important priority meal that utilises 30% of our total daily intake.

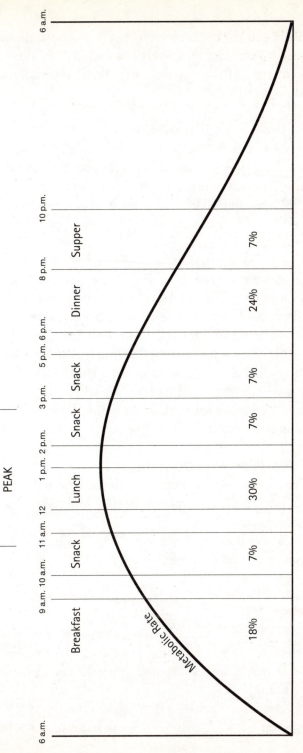

Distribution of food (percentages) in relation to metabolic rate within a 24-hour period.

An intake of 1200 to 1400 calories eaten in seven small meals during the day is utilised far more effectively than one 1200 calorie intake at night. At that time of the day we are 'parked', sedentary and going NOWHERE.

Breakfast time – 6.00–9.00 a.m.

Breakfast is the foundation stone of our seven daily intakes. We must eat breakfast. The timing of breakfast is dictated by the time we rise each morning, but you must, if possible, eat no later than 9.00 a.m. Between 6.00 a.m. and 10.00 a.m. our metabolic rate is on the rise. Eating breakfast early kicks the metabolic rate, which has dropped during the night, into action.

To say that you skip breakfast because you don't have time is a poor excuse. The obvious solution is to rise 10 minutes earlier, and making this small change to your schedule will reward you with a balanced day. When I had to travel to the city for an early lecture, I left home at 6.00 a.m. to beat the traffic and travelled with a small basket I had packed the night before (a two-minute job). Having reached my destination I parked in a safe location overlooking floral gardens. I relaxed in the knowledge I was on time and had a car park, and could enjoy my breakfast unrushed while listening to my radio. What could have been a stressful situation became quality time out.

Morning-tea time – 10.00 a.m.

The time you eat your breakfast will determine what you eat for morning tea. If you eat breakfast between 6.00 a.m. and 7.00 a.m., select from box one on page 72.

If your breakfast is eaten closer to 9.00 a.m., you only need a small top-up so you will select from box two.

Lunch time – 12.00–1.00 p.m.

Lunch is the most important meal of the day.

Between 11.00 a.m. and 2.00 p.m. our appetite is most stimulated and our digestive system is at its most efficient. It makes sense to consume our largest intake at this time, when the energy can be utilised rather than stored as fat.

Many women argue that they don't have time to eat a large lunch and save up their intake for dinner. I speak to groups of women every day, and over the years I have heard every excuse in the book for why women don't have time to fit regular meals into their lives. I find very few of those reasons valid. Create a routine, it isn't that difficult when you put your mind to it, and you will feel the benefits immediately.

I would like you to consider the possibility that your snack lunches may well be partly the cause of your weight problem. The lunch choices of some people horrify me, and it is no wonder that they cave in at late afternoon when all they had for lunch was a yoghurt and fruit or a cup of fat-free diet soup. If you want to achieve weight loss, don't procrastinate, get on with it and make the necessary changes.

Understand that a larger lunch does not have to be a cooked meal, such as a casserole or a roast dinner. It is simply the difference between, as an example, a sandwich with one thin processed cheese slice and a BIG, filled to the brim, chicken, avocado, salad and sprout sandwich that you have to attack from the corner as it is too large to bite into. Trust me on this one.

Afternoon snacks – Double top-up at 2.00 p.m. and 3.30–4.00 p.m.

Afternoons are the most vulnerable period of the day – the time we are most at risk of over-eating. Our metabolic rate is gradually declining and mid-way through the afternoon, between 3.00 p.m. and 4.00 p.m., we begin to experience a drop in energy and mental concentration. This is due to the drop in our serotonin and endorphin levels that we discussed in *Hormones on the Rampage* earlier. To maintain these levels we are going to position two planned snacks into the afternoon slot.

Let us say that you have eaten a large sandwich at lunch that will satisfy you if given a chance. Do not 'tag' a piece of fruit to your sandwich, but rather let your lunch go down, and then around 2.00 p.m. eat your first snack, your piece of fruit. It takes 20 minutes for the sense of satiety to kick in, and you will feel fuller if you eat the fruit later. I hate big gaps in my eating. When lunch and snacks are eaten in one sitting it can seem a very long time until dinner!

As children we were not allowed to snack between meals. 'Wait, your dinner is nearly ready – a snack will spoil your appetite!' We sat down to dinner hungry, scoffed the meal, and then asked, 'What's for pudding?' Spoil our dinner! Today that is exactly what I want. Now I enjoy my dinner far more when I am not 'starving', I eat more slowly, am aware of what I am eating, and don't overeat or continue eating after dinner.

I find that women who try to brave it out through the afternoon without having a snack are those most at risk of over-eating into the night. They hold out until they get home, then one mouthful and WHAM – they eat until they drop. Hunger is cumulative, and it is my belief that we need to eat on the 'other side of hunger'. By this I mean that rather than holding out until you are hungry, which you will find is usually within a specific time frame, eat prior to that time.

Let me give you an example – if you find you are ravenous at 4.00 p.m. every afternoon, and that once you start eating you can't stop, you need to bring that snack forward until 3.15 p.m. or 3.30 p.m., regardless of whether you feel hungry or not. The theory that we should listen to our bodies and wait for the physiological urge of hunger to cut in before we eat is, to me, a faulty proposition. Waiting until I am hungry leads me into a danger zone. Whereas one slice of toast may have sufficed at 3.30 p.m. (when I wasn't all that hungry) waiting until 4.00 p.m. when my hunger did cut in meant I was more likely to eat the LOAF!

One of my members who had reached her goal weight, was out and about shopping with her husband. It was getting late in the afternoon and she was anxious to get home for her afternoon snack. When it came to 4.00 o'clock, and he suddenly pulled into a building-supply yard, her patience snapped.

'I want to go home,' she demanded. 'Now!'

'Why?' he asked, 'we are here, and it will only take a couple of minutes.'

'I don't care if it is only one minute – IT IS TIME FOR MY TOAST AND I WANT IT NOW!'

They went home.

Dinner time – 6.00–7.00 p.m. (no later than 8.00 p.m.)
Time for change.

Change your carbohydrate intake. Eat carbohydrate with dinner three nights a week only.

Change your dinner time so that you are eating earlier.

Change your heavy dinner for a lighter meal.

How? Let us deal with each change individually.

1. Change your carbohydrate intake at night

**A key element of the Middle-Age Spread Diet
is to restrict the use of carbohydrates at dinner
to THREE nights a week only.**

You can select any three nights to use your carbohydrates but realise that three nights are the maximum. You can have fewer carbohydrate nights if you wish. This means that there will be at least four dinners in your week that you will serve to yourself **without** a carbohydrate, and this includes breads, rice, pasta and potato as well as all the other foods listed in the Carbohydrate list.

The three nights that carbohydrates are permitted you may select ONE or TWO extra Carbohydrates in addition to the daily allowance. If you aren't particularly hungry and are using lots of vegetables, then you will probably find one Carbohydrate is sufficient.

Will this change be difficult to achieve? NO.

I usually select my carbohydrate nights based on the recipe. Obviously a filo-pastry dish or a pasta recipe can only be used on my carbohydrate nights, and I always include one roast-dinner meal in my week with my roast potato. The other nights I happily grill chops, cook stir-fries, chargrill chicken and fish, and surround them with mountains of freshly cooked vegetables. On these nights I still serve the potato/rice/pasta to my family. Don't worry, nobody notices and nobody cares that you haven't got any carbohydrate on your plate.

They're too busy enjoying their own meals. It's an easy way to integrate the food plan into your everyday cooking.

**Am I cooking separate meals? Definitely not –
the only difference is in the dishing up.**

2. Eating dinner earlier

Arriving home late, or waiting for your family to fight their way home through the traffic, can necessitate late evening meals. Waiting for dinner can cause us to begin picking, and by the time dinner arrives we are really not all that hungry – but we still eat the big dinner. I appreciate it isn't always possible to eat earlier if you want to share the meal with family members, but sometimes late eating becomes more of a habit than a necessity.

Over-eating a huge meal at dinner, especially if it is late, not only causes weight gain but also sleep disturbances, digestion and elimination problems, and can contribute to night sweats.

3. Lighten up!

Dinner for many of us has traditionally been the largest meal of the day, a habit that is not in harmony with our metabolic rate, which is in decline at a time when many of us are consuming our largest intake of calories. Meat, three vegetables and heaps of potatoes were acceptable when we were younger, but at middle-age we can no longer process this calorie saturation late at night. Our bodies are now preparing for sleep, and even though we may stay up late, it is against our natural rhythms.

Portions
Portions
Portions

There is no getting away from the fact that our meals have been getting bigger. When I am asked the question 'Why haven't I lost weight this week when I have cooked your recipes?' I often find the answer is portions. If there are only two of you at home and you have cooked my recipe for four servings AND there is nothing left then you have effectively eaten two servings each.

Watch your portions!

To gain maximum satisfaction with a smaller intake you might find this suggestion helpful. Eat the protein on your plate first. Protein stimulates the production of the appetite-regulating hormones. It is possible that by doing this your body will receive the signals that you are full sooner and prevents you from over-eating. I always used to eat my vegetables first, followed by my carbohydrate and finished with my protein. Reversing this order has made a difference to my level of satiety.

After dinner dessert/supper/snack

Home alone and in charge of the fridge and pantry!

Late night is sometimes the only time we get to be alone, in peace and quiet, and it is then that we may feel tempted to have a little reward. In our food plan we have allocated a late-night snack, and this is something to look forward to and enjoy.

Many of the women I speak to have two jobs or work night shifts and don't get home until the family is tucked up in bed. Dinner seems a long time ago, they have worked hard and are now entering a new time slot. Eating late is not advisable, but going to bed on an empty grumbling stomach is unsettling. Hot stewed apple and yoghurt is ideal for settling you down, or maybe try an oldie-but-a-goodie – hot milk with a dash of vanilla essence and a sprinkle of nutmeg. It's nature's natural sleeping remedy.

In the next section I am going to take you progressively through three stages of the Middle-Age Spread Diet. We will begin with lists of the **Daily Food Allowances**, which will allow you to familiarise yourself with the basic foods available. These are the building blocks for each day.

Lists are essential but often confusing, leaving us with a jumble of foods and no clear idea of how to utilise them correctly. I have, therefore, followed the Food Allowance Lists with **Meal-by-Meal** suggestions that present you with lots of choices, which are interchangeable, depending on your personal preferences.

To consolidate this information I have prepared three weeks of **Food Planners**, which will talk you through **21 days of delicious meals**. For those of you who are on the run, and just want to get a meal on the table, I have a special **On-the-Run Planner**, which will be useful for busy weeks.

Daily Food Allowances

BREAKFAST PACKAGE

All foods in each breakfast are additional to the daily allowances in other meals.

PLUS

LUNCH, DINNER AND SNACKS

For these meals you have the following daily food allowances.

FOOD GROUPS	A	B	C
Proteins	2	2	2
Carbohydrates*	3	4	4
Fats	3	3	4
Milk/Yoghurt	4	4	4
Fruits	3	3	4
Bits on the Side	2	2	2
Vegetables/Salads	UNLIMITED	UNLIMITED	UNLIMITED

* Three nights per week you'll be allowed one or two extra Carbohydrates for dinner (refer page 59).

PLUS each week you can select
FOUR SHEER INDULGENCES.

As you can see there is plenty of food available each and every day. To provide our energy intake and maintain good health we need to incorporate, in the right proportions, a variety of foods from the above groups. Eliminating one food while over-compensating on another does not equate to balanced nutrition. I believe it is easier to follow the Middle-Age Spread Diet if you establish the pattern that works best for you and leave it in place most of the time. Once you understand how the day is laid out, it will simply become the way that you eat.

Now let us begin with the Breakfast Package.

Breakfast Package (A, B and C)

Each breakfast package is a complete meal and you don't have to take it out of your daily allowances. Remember each package is complete and you cannot interchange part of one for part of another.

All breakfasts are additional to all the other allocated daily allowances.

To keep life simple, and to get you off to the right start in the mornings, I have listed three quick breakfast packages to choose from, but you can select any of the other options from the list on page 71.

Let's begin our day and select one of the following:

Cereal and Fruit Breakfast

Select the cereal of your choice

1 fruit serving from the list on pages 63–64
1/2 cup milk or 1/4 yoghurt
Tea/Coffee

3/4 cup	1/2 cup	1/4 cup
Cornflakes	All Bran	Rolled Oats
Puffed Wheat	Bran Flakes	
Ricies	Light and Tasty	2 pieces of
	Special K	Weet-Bix
	Sultana Bran	Bran-Bix

or

Something on Toast

1 slice wholemeal toast, spread with 1 teaspoon butter served topped with **one** of the following:
1 egg, poached or boiled
100 grams baked beans
65 grams cottage cheese
25 grams cheddar cheese
Tea/Coffee

or

Fresh Fruit Salad

Select 3 fruit servings of your choice from list pages 63–64.
Serve with 1/4 cup yoghurt
Tea/Coffee

or

Select any breakfast of your choice from page 71.

Protein

Choose **ONE** protein serving at lunch and **ONE** protein serving at dinner. Each day select your protein quantities using your designated rating, A, B, or C. Proteins in the Restricted List are high in cholesterol and calories. Limit these to no more than **FIVE** servings in total per week.

		Serving Size	
Preferred Proteins	**A**	**B**	**C**
Bacon, lean	2 rashers	2 rashers	2 rashers
Baked beans	170 grams	190 grams	210 grams
Cheese, feta	50 grams	50 grams	55 grams
Cheese, ricotta	100 grams	110 grams	120 grams
Chicken (cooked and skinned)	100 grams	110 grams	120 grams
Cottage cheese	125 grams	140 grams	160 grams
Egg and bacon	1 egg and 1 bacon rasher	1 egg and 1 bacon rasher	2 eggs and 1 bacon rasher
Eggs	2 eggs	2 eggs	2 eggs
Fish			
• all fresh and smoked fish (cooked)	120 grams	130 grams	140 grams
• canned salmon, tuna, sardines	100 grams	110 grams	120 grams
• lobster, crayfish, shrimp, crab,	120 grams	130 grams	140 grams
• mussels, oysters, scallops,	120 grams	130 grams	140 grams
• calamari, whitebait	120 grams	130 grams	140 grams
Turkey	100 grams	110 grams	120 grams
Venison	100 grams	110 grams	120 grams

Restricted Proteins – Limit to 5 servings per week

	A	B	C
Beef (cooked) steak, mince, roast, silverside	100 grams	110 grams	120 grams
Cheese • blue, brie, camembert, cheddar, edam, gouda, Gruyère, mascarpone, mozzarella	50 grams	50 grams	55 grams
Ham	100 grams	110 grams	120 grams
Lamb (cooked) • fillet, roast • chops	100 grams 2 chops	110 grams 2 chops	120 grams 3 chops
Liver/kidney/tripe	100 grams	110 grams	120 grams
Pork (cooked) • fillet, roast • chop	100 grams 1 small	110 grams 1 small	120 grams 1 medium
Sausages/Frankfurters	2 small	2 small	2 small
Veal	100 grams	110 grams	120 grams

Protein Note Weights listed are cooked weights – add approximately 20 grams to the raw weight to allow for shrinkage.

Proteins for Vegetarian Meals

	A	B	C
Baked beans	170 grams	190 grams	210 grams
*Cheese • brie, blue, camembert, cheddar, edam, gouda, Gruyère, mascarpone, mozzarella	50 grams	50 grams	55 grams
Cheese • feta • ricotta	50 grams 100 grams	50 grams 110 grams	55 grams 120 grams

cont.

Proteins for Vegetarian Meals

	A	B	C
Cottage cheese	125 grams	140 grams	160 grams
Eggs	2 eggs	2 eggs	2 eggs
Fish			
• all fresh and smoked fish (cooked)	120 grams	130 grams	140 grams
• canned, salmon, tuna, sardines	100 grams	110 grams	120 grams
• lobster, crayfish, shrimp, crab, mussels, oysters, scallops, calamari, whitebait	120 grams	130 grams	140 grams
Nuts, raw			
• almonds	24 nuts	26 nuts	28 nuts
• brazils	7 nuts	8 nuts	9 nuts
• cashews	15 nuts	16 nuts	17 nuts
• peanuts	15 nuts	16 nuts	17 nuts
• pine nuts	3 tablespoons	3 tablespoons	4 tablespoons
• pistachio	18 nuts	19 nuts	20 nuts
• walnuts	10 halves	11 halves	12 halves
Pulses (cooked)			
• broad beans, chickpeas, haricot beans, kidney beans, lentils, lima beans, split peas	180 grams	210 grams	240 grams
Quark	125 grams	140 grams	160 grams
Tofu	240 grams	260 grams	280 grams

Vegetarian Protein Notes * Cheese is a Restricted Protein – limit it to no more than five servings a week. Cottage cheese, feta and ricotta, however, are not restricted and you can use them in the listed portions as many times a week as you wish.

It is important when making the decision to give up eating meat that you do not overlook the fact that you still need to have an adequate supply of protein. Simply eating vegetables on their own will not provide all the amino acids necessary for good health. Make sure you use your three carbohydrate allowances each day and that you select the additional Carbohydrate three nights a week to ensure you have a balanced food plan.

Carbohydrates

The number of servings below are to be used only for lunches or snacks.
Each day select the number of servings based on your A B C rating.

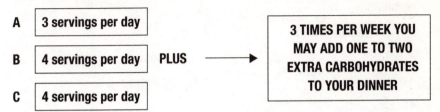

A	3 servings per day	
B	4 servings per day	**PLUS** →
C	4 servings per day	

3 TIMES PER WEEK YOU MAY ADD ONE TO TWO EXTRA CARBOHYDRATES TO YOUR DINNER

	Serving Size
Bread, whole grain/wholemeal	1 slice
Breadcrumbs	2 tablespoons
Bread roll/Bagel	$^1/_2$ medium roll
Burghul wheat (dry)	$^1/_4$ cup
Cereal	$^1/_4$ cup
Couscous (dry)	$^1/_4$ cup
Crackers	2 large or 4 small
Crumpet	1
Digestive biscuit	1 plain biscuit
Filo pastry	1 sheet
Flour	$^1/_4$ cup
Hamburger bun	$^1/_2$ medium bun
Kumara (cooked)	100–120 grams
Noodles, Udon/Hokkien	50 grams fresh
Panini	$^1/_2$ medium
Pasta (uncooked), orzo	$^1/_4$ cup
• cannelloni	3 tubes
• fettucine, lasagne, macaroni, spaghetti	30 grams dried or 50 grams fresh

cont.

	Serving Size
Pita pocket	
• small	1
• medium	$^1/_2$
Popcorn (plain, popped)	1 cup
Polenta	3 tablespoons
Potato (cooked)	100–120 grams
Rice (cooked)	$^1/_2$ cup
Rice (uncooked)	$^1/_4$ cup
Rice cake	1 large
Rice wafers	10 thin, small
Rolled oats	$^1/_4$ cup
Sweetcorn	1 small ear or $^1/_2$ cup canned
Taro (cooked)	120 grams
Tortillas	1 small
Yams (cooked)	120 grams

Carbohydrate Note To list all the breads and carbohydrates available would be unrealistic. Therefore, to provide a general guideline when choosing your product, do not exceed 80 calories per carbohydrate, and one bread serving must not weigh more than 30 grams per serving.

Fats
Each day select the number of servings based on your A B C rating.

A	3 servings per day

B	3 servings per day

C	4 servings per day

	Serving Size
Avocado	1 tablespoon
Butter	1 teaspoon (5 grams)
Cream cheese	1 teaspoon
Hummus	1 tablespoon
Margarine	1 teaspoon
Mayonnaise	1 teaspoon
Oil • avocado, canola, flaxseed, olive, peanut, safflower, sesame, soy, sunflower, walnut	1 teaspoon
Olivio	1 teaspoon
Peanut butter	1 teaspoon
Pesto	1 teaspoon
Sour cream	1 tablespoon
Tahini	1 teaspoon
Vinaigrette (refer page 221)	4 teaspoons

Know Your Fats Fats provide calories and, nutritionally, very little else. One gram of fat has 9 calories compared with 4.5 calories per gram for protein and carbohydrate.

Fats can be broken down into four main categories:

Saturated	butter, cream, coconut oil, coconut milk, beef, cheese, pork
Trans Fatty Acids	margarine, vegetable shortening, many fast foods, deep-fried chips
Monounsaturated oils	olive, canola, peanut
Polyunsaturated oils	corn, soy bean, safflower, fish

Oils provide essential fatty acids (EFAs), which nourish dry skin, hair and mucous membranes, aid in natural hormone production and transport calcium into the soft tissues.

Many supermarket oils are highly refined causing them to oxidise easily when heated, which can contribute to arterial plaque. Plant oils such as olive, canola and soy are considered the most stable oils.

Milk products/yoghurt

Each day you may select **FOUR** servings.

A | **4 servings per day**

B | **4 servings per day**

C | **4 servings per day**

	Serving Size
Milk, dairy	
• Trim, buttermilk, Calci-Trim, Lite Blue	1/2 cup
Milk, non-dairy	
• coconut (Lite)	1/4 cup
• soy (Lite)	1/2 cup
Milk powder	
• coconut	1 tablespoon
• dairy (Lite)	2 tablespoons
Yoghurt	
• plain or fruit	1/4 cup
• soy	1/4 cup
Other	
• cottage cheese	4 tablespoons
• custard, commercial	1/4 cup

Milk and Yoghurt Notes Milk products provide protein, vitamins and minerals. Milk and yoghurt are recommended for your calcium intake. Avoid using full-cream milk.

If you drink milk with your tea or coffee, calculate your average daily usage. 1 cup tea/coffee uses approximately 2 tablespoons of milk, so 4 cups would use 8 tablespoons = 1 serving.

Measurement Guide

1/2 cup	=	125 ml	1/4 cup	=	4 tablespoons
1 cup	=	250 ml	1 tablespoon	=	3 teaspoons

Fruits
Each day select the number of servings based on your A B C rating.

A | 3 servings per day

B | 3 servings per day

C | 4 servings per day

	Serving Size
Apple	1
Apricots	2
Banana, small	1
Berries • blackberries, blueberries, boysenberries, raspberries	$^3/_4$ cup
Cherries	12
Feijoas	2
Grapefruit	1
Grapes	12
Kiwifruit	2
Mandarins	2
Mango, small	1
Melon	1 cup
Nashi pear	1
Nectarine	1
Orange	1
Pawpaw	1 cup
Passionfruit	2
Peach	1

cont.

	Serving Size
Pear	1
Persimmon, small	1
Pineapple, fresh	1 cup
Plums	2
Strawberries	1 cup
Tamarillos	2
Tangelo/Tangerine	1
Watermelon	1 cup
Dried Fruits	
• apricot halves	4
• craisins	2 tablespoons
• dates	4
• figs	2
• prunes	2
• raisins	2 tablespoons
• sultanas	2 tablespoons
Canned Fruits	
• All canned fruit, drained	1/2 cup
Crystallized Fruits	
• cherries	2 tablespoons
• ginger	2 tablespoons
• pineapple	2 tablespoons
Stewed Fruits	
• All sweetened stewed fruit	1/2 cup
• Apple sauce	1/2 cup
• Rhubarb stewed with sugar	1/2 cup

Fruit Notes There is no great advantage in using diabetic canned fruit or fruit canned in fruit juice as you will be required to drain it anyway.

Use fresh fruit when available, but if you choose canned fruit always select on the basis of your personal preference.

Vegetables

A

B

```
┌─────────────────────────────────┐
│           UNLIMITED             │
│         As listed below         │
│                                 │
└─────────────────────────────────┘
```

C

Asparagus	Cucumber
Beans, green	Eggplant
Bean sprouts, alfalfa, broccoli, mung, radish, snowpea	Leeks
	Lettuce
Beetroot	Mushrooms
Bok choy	Onions
	Parsnips
Broccoli	Peas
Brussels sprouts	Pumpkin
Cabbage, red, savoy, Chinese	Radishes
Capsicums, red, green, yellow	Rhubarb*
	Silverbeet
Carrots	Spinach
Cauliflower	Spring onions
Celery	Swedes
Choko	Tomatoes
Courgettes	Watercress

```
┌──────────────────────────────┐
│  The starchy vegetables      │
│  listed below are            │
│  carbohydrates and are not   │
│  part of this free vegetable │
│  list.                       │
│                              │
│         Potato               │
│         Kumara               │
│        Sweetcorn             │
│          Taro                │
│           Yam                │
└──────────────────────────────┘
```

Vegetable Notes Don't confuse eating vegetables with HAVING to eat 'rabbit food' in order to lose weight. You will lose weight without ever biting into a raw carrot. Eat vegetables for good health not weight loss. They provide many essential minerals and vitamins, and the consumption of vegetables has been linked to the prevention of some cancers.

Hot vegetables are more filling than salads, and it is recommended that you serve hot vegetables with your dinner and lunch if possible. Use salads as a side dish.

* Rhubarb is listed as a vegetable – when sweetened it is treated as a fruit serving.

Bits on the Side

Each day you may select **TWO** servings.

A | 2 servings per day |

B | 2 servings per day |

C | 2 servings per day |

	Serving Size
Chutney	1 tablespoon
Cocoa	2 teaspoons
Coconut, desiccated	2 teaspoons
Cordial, Roses Lime	1 tablespoon
Cream, whipped	1 tablespoon
Custard powder	2 teaspoons
Egg whites	2
Flour/Cornflour/Arrowroot	2 teaspoons
Honey	2 teaspoons
Horlicks	1 tablespoon
Jam/Marmalade	2 teaspoons
Lemon curd	2 teaspoons
Liquor/Alcohol	1 teaspoon
Milo	1 teaspoon
Nuts • almonds, cashews, pine nuts, walnuts	1 tablespoon
Olives, black/green	4
Parmesan cheese	2 teaspoons
Peanut butter	1 teaspoon
Pickles, onions/dill/gherkins	2

cont.

	Serving Size
Relish	1 tablespoon
Sauces • black bean, char siu, teriyaki, tomato	2 tablespoons
Seeds • linseed, pumpkin, sesame, sunflower	1 tablespoon
Sugar	2 teaspoons
Syrup • golden, maple	2 teaspoons
Tomato paste/purée	2 tablespoons

Bits on the Side Note Two little treats a day.

Use your Bits on the Side wherever you wish – but remember there are only two choices per day. Remember when you have used them.

Sheer Indulgence
EACH WEEK you may choose **FOUR** servings.

A | 4 servings per week |

B | 4 servings per week |

C | 4 servings per week |

		Serving size
From the bar	Beer	1 can
	Cider, sweet	1 glass (177 ml)
	Liqueur	1 glass (28 ml)
	Port	1 glass (55 ml)
	Sherry, sweet or dry	1 glass (55 ml)
	Spirits	1 double nip (40 ml) or 2 single nips (20 ml)
	Wine • sparkling, red/rosé, dry white	1 glass (104 ml)
Non-alcoholic	Fruit juice	1/2 cup (125 ml)
	Ginger-beer	1 cup (250ml)
	Soft drinks, regular	1 cup (250 ml)
Frozen confections	Ice block, not chocolate	1
	Ice-cream, regular	1/4 cup
	Yoghurt, frozen	1/4 cup
Sweet treats	Chocolates, fancy, filled	3
	Jelly, made with water	1/2 cup
	Jellybeans	12
	Marshmallows, pink/white	6
Miscellaneous	Avocado	1/4
	Cream, whipped	3 tablespoons
	Egg	1 (for baking only)

Sheer Indulgence Note If you wish you may use the FOUR SERVINGS on ONE occasion. Just remember not to have any more for the rest of the week.

Herbs, spices, sauces and beverages – unlimited

Not only do herbs and spices add flavour to our meals but they are healthy. Some spices, such as chilli, cumin, turmeric, cardamom, cinnamon, mustard seed and black pepper stimulate digestion and can lift the metabolic rate by up to 25%.

Herbs

Basil

Chives

Garlic

Mint

Parsley – a must – a great diuretic

Rosemary

Thyme

Spices to include in your food plan

Cardamom

Chilli – adds some fire

Cinnamon

Cumin

Curry

Ginger

Paprika

Turmeric

Vanilla – (Vanilla Sugar refer page 233)

Condiments and sauces

Mint sauce

Mustard

Soy sauce

Sweet chilli sauce

Vegemite/Marmite

Vinegar

- balsamic
- malt
- rice
- tarragon
- wine

Worcestershire sauce

Fresh adds zest

Red and green chillies – hot as!

Lemons

Root ginger

Beverages

Coffee, tea, green tea and herbal tea, mineral water, soda water, water

Excite the taste-buds! Think about biting into a lemon and what happens? You activate the taste-buds and you salivate. Add lemon and orange zest to salad, desserts and stir-fries.

Be Fresh! Freshly grated ginger and crushed garlic taste totally different to the commercially prepared varieties. Try grating ginger on fresh fruit salads and adding it to stir-fries.

The Complete Picture – A List

FOOD GROUP	Breakfast	Snack	Lunch	Snack	Snack	Dinner	After-Dinner
ONE Breakfast Package	1						
TWO Protein			1			1	
THREE Carbohydrate			2		1	Carb free	
THREE Fats			1		1	1	
FOUR Milk/Yoghurt		1			1		1
THREE Fruits		1		1			1
TWO Bits on the Side	Optional Placement						
UNLIMITED Vegetables/Salads	No Limit						
EXTRA CARBOHYDRATE Three times per week						2	

UNUSED
1 Milk/Yoghurt
for Tea/Coffee

Meal by Meal
Learning to put it together

It's as easy as looking at a menu and selecting your choice for each meal.
Read through, make your selection, prepare it and enjoy.

The Breakfast package
Eat breakfast before 9.00 a.m.
Every morning choose one of the following:

Cereal and Fruit
Cereal of your choice (refer page 55)
1 fruit serving
and $1/2$ cup milk or $1/4$ cup yoghurt

Egg on Toast
1 egg, boiled or poached
1 slice wholegrain toast spread with 1 teaspoon butter

Fresh Fruit Salad
Select 3 fruit servings and chop into large chunks. Or try a mix of 6 half servings e.g. $1/2$ banana, $1/2$ apple, $1/2$ orange, 1 kiwifruit, 1 tablespoon raisins and 2 dried apricot halves. Place in a large bowl and top with a swirl of yoghurt ($1/4$ cup).

Hot Almond Latte
Heat 1 cup milk in a small pot.
Into a latte bowl or large mug spoon 2 teaspoons ground almonds, $1/2$ teaspoon raw sugar and a sprinkle of cardamom. Pour hot milk over and stir well to combine.

Sesame Cottage Cheese on Toast
Toast 1 slice wholemeal bread. Top with tomato slices and cottage cheese (50 grams). Sprinkle with 1 teaspoon toasted sesame seeds.

Coffee, Walnut and Date Smoothie
Blend together 1 cup milk, 1 teaspoon coffee granules, 2 dried dates, 2 walnut halves and 1 teaspoon honey. Serve frothed in a tall glass.

Green Velvet Smoothie
Blend together 1 cup milk, $1/2$ banana, 2 teaspoons Spirulina, 1 teaspoon honey and ice cubes. Serve frothed in a tall glass.

Breakfast Pancakes with Lemon Honey (refer page 155)
Bircher Muesli (refer page 157)
A Symphony of Grains, Seeds and Fruit (refer page 154)
Gingered Fruit Compote (refer page 158)

Morning-tea time

Remember – timing is everything.

Keeping in mind our scallop effect of eating at regular intervals, your choice will be based on what time you ate breakfast.

10.00 a.m.

If you ate breakfast between 6.00 a.m. and 7.00 a.m.

> You may select 1 Fruit and 1 Milk/Yoghurt
> e.g.
> 1 fruit serving and ¼ cup yoghurt
> Try 1 orange cut into slices and drizzled with fruit yoghurt
> 1 peach cut in 2 halves, lightly grilled, served with yoghurt
> 1 apple, baked and served with yoghurt
> 1 nectarine, sliced and served with 50 grams cottage cheese
> Tea or Coffee

If you ate breakfast between 7.00 a.m. and 8.30 a.m.

> You may select 1 Fruit serving
> e.g.
> 1 apple
> 2 kiwifruit
> 1 small banana
> 4 dried apricot halves
> ½ cup stewed apple
> ½ cup canned fruit, drained
> Tea or coffee

If you ate breakfast after 8.30 a.m.

> Enjoy a cup of tea or coffee and wait until lunchtime for your next intake.
> Remember – try to eat your lunch between 12.00 and 1.00 p.m.

Lunch time

Each day try to eat your lunch between 12.00 noon and 1.00 p.m. Using the allowances listed below, you can enjoy all these delicious lunches.

Or you can create your own meal by using the Daily Food Allowances on pages 56–69.

2 Carbohydrates	1 Protein	1 Fat	Unlimited Salad or Vegetables	Additional: Milk/Yoghurt, Bits on the Side

The recommended pattern for lunch, which I have used here, is that you always use:

2 Carbohydrate servings, e.g. 2 breads, or 200 grams potato, or 1 cup rice.

Add 1 Fat of your choice, e.g. 1 teaspoon butter, or 1 tablespoon avocado.

Fill or top your Carbohydrate with 1 serving of Protein, e.g. 2 eggs, or 100 grams chicken.

Use as many salad greens, sprouts, tomatoes, etc. as you wish – make it a lot.

Let's make lunch.

The Big Sandwich

Use 2 slices of wholemeal bread and spread with

BLAT	1 tablespoon avocado. Fill with 2 grilled rashers bacon, sliced tomato and lots of mixed greens.
Curried Egg	1 teaspoon butter. Fill with 2 hard-boiled eggs mashed with ½ teaspoon curry powder, 1 spring onion, chopped parsley, salt and pepper. Stir in 1 tablespoon crunchy mixed sprouts.
Smoked Salmon	1 teaspoon cream cheese. Fill with 100 grams smoked salmon, thin cucumber slices, chopped dill, salt and pepper.
Roasted Vegetable	1 tablespoon hummus. Fill with 50 grams mozzarella, and *Roasted Vegetables* (refer page 217).

Pita Pockets

You might like to toast a pocket to transform it into a crisp shell.

Use 1 medium pita pocket OR 2 small pita pockets, line with lettuce and fill with one of these combinations.

Cottage Cheese	125 grams cottage cheese. Chunky Salad: mix together 1 teaspoon mayonnaise, 2 tablespoons natural yoghurt, chopped tomato, cucumber, parsley, spring onion, salt and pepper. Spoon in alternate layers of cottage cheese and chunky salad.
Tuna Mayonnaise	Mix together 100 grams tuna, 2 sun-dried tomatoes, 1 teaspoon mayonnaise, squeeze lemon juice, salt and pepper.
Chicken Caesar	Mix together 100 grams cooked chicken, squeeze lemon juice, 1 teaspoon mayonnaise, 2 tablespoons yoghurt, 1 teaspoon Dijon mustard, salt and pepper. Fill pocket with chicken mixture, top with tomato chunks and 2 teaspoons shaved Parmesan (optional).
Turkish Lamb	100 grams cooked lamb, tomato chunks, salt, pepper and top with 1 tablespoon hummus sprinkled with fresh mint.

Something on Toast

Use 2 slices wholemeal bread, toasted, and 1 Fat spread of your choice topped with one of these combinations.

Salmon	*Chunky Salmon Pâté* (refer page 174).
Herbed Scrambled Eggs	2 eggs, scrambled. Stir in chopped chives or oregano.
Baked Beans	170 grams baked beans cooked with finely chopped celery, seasoned with black pepper and topped with chopped parsley.
Poached Egg with Smoked Salmon and Asparagus	Add asparagus, 1 poached egg and 50 grams smoked salmon. Season with salt, ground black pepper and snipped chives.

Bread Rolls
Use 1 medium bread roll or 1 small bagel spread with

Ham Bagel	1 teaspoon butter. Fill with 100 grams shaved ham, topped with grainy seed mustard, cucumber and tomato slices, alfalfa and lettuce.
Burger	*Gourmet Chicken Burger* (refer page 169) – this recipe uses half a fruit so reduce your afternoon snack to $1/2$ a fruit serving.

Going Crackers
Cold Meat and Chutney	Use 4 Ryvitas or 2 Carbohydrates of your choice spread with 1 teaspoon butter, topped with 100 grams cold meat, alfalfa, 1 tablespoon chutney, sliced tomato, salt and pepper.

A Bit of Crumpet
Poached Eggs	Toast 2 crumpets and lightly spread with 1 teaspoon butter. Top with 2 poached eggs, salt, pepper and chopped parsley.

Filo Pastry
Tomato, Basil and Ricotta Flan (refer page 197).

Panini
Toasted Cheese and Ham	Use 1 medium panini, split and spread with 1 teaspoon pesto. Fill with 50 grams ham, 25 grams grated cheese and slices of tomato. Toast under grill or in sandwich press.

Pasta
Chicken and Corn Pasta Salad (refer page 168).

Verde Fettucine with Ham and Mascarpone Sauce (refer page 192).

Grains
Burghul Wheat	*Vegetable Tabbouleh* (refer page 216), toss with Protein of your choice e.g. 50 grams feta, or 100 grams chicken.
Couscous	*Arabian Nights Chicken Salad* (refer page 164).

Potato/Kumara

Use 200 grams baked potato **or** kumara and top with one of these combinations.

Cottage cheese   125 grams cottage cheese, chunks of tomato, cucumber, red pepper. Sprinkle with aduki beans and alfalfa. Drizzle with dressing of your choice (refer page 221).

Tuna/Salmon   100 grams tuna/salmon mixed with 1 tablespoon sour cream. Fold in chopped spring onion, parsley, salt and ground black pepper.

Fritters   *Potato Fritters* (refer page 215).

Chicken   *Smoked chicken with Walnut and Potato Salad* (refer page 163).

Rice

Sushi   *Sesame Tuna Sushi* (refer page 181), or you can purchase prepared sushi – 6 pieces.

Sweetcorn

Sweetcorn Fritters with a Ginger and Chilli Sauce (refer page 191).

Lunch can be served with tea or coffee.

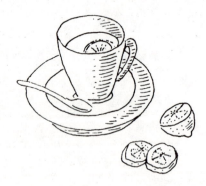

Afternoon-tea time

Each afternoon select either two snacks or one combined snack as shown below. Remember this is a vulnerable time of the day – make sure you use your snacks daily.

Between 2.00 p.m. and 4.00 p.m.

2.00 p.m.

You may select 1 Fruit serving

Refer to Fruit list on pages 63–64.

e.g.
1 apple
1 orange
1 pear
1 peach
2 kiwifruit
2 plums
4 dried dates

4.00 p.m.

You may select the following allowances:

1 Carbohydrate, 1 Fat, 1 Bit on Side, 1 Milk/ Yoghurt. Put allowances together and enjoy, for example:

1 slice wholemeal bread, toasted, spread with 1 teaspoon butter and 2 teaspoons jam.

2 Ryvitas spread with 1 teaspoon pesto topped with 50 grams cottage cheese and 2 sliced gherkins.

1 slice grainy bread spread with 1 table-spoon avocado, topped with sliced tomatoes and alfalfa.

1 slice *Cinnamon Toast* (refer page 233).

OR

Combine allowances and use between 3.00 p.m. and 4.00 p.m.

You may select 1 Fruit, 1 Carbohydrate, 1 Fat, 1 Bit on the Side, 1 Milk/Yoghurt and, if you wish, one of your Sheer Indulgences to combine and create the following afternoon snacks.

Banana Split	Use 1 sheet filo pastry brushed with 1 teaspoon butter. Fold sheet in half, place banana on sheet, and roll. Bake at 210°C for 5–8 min. Split and drizzle with 1/4 cup yoghurt and 1 teaspoon honey.
2 slices *Maple Fruit and Nut Loaf*	(refer page 234)
Blueberry Muffin	(refer page 231)
1 slice toast	Spread with 1 teaspoon peanut butter and topped with 1/2 mashed banana.

Afternoon tea can be served with tea or coffee.

Dinner time

Try to eat your dinner between 6.00 p.m. and 7.00 p.m. and no later than 8.00 p.m. Each day you have the allowances listed below available to you for dinner. You may create your own menu from the Daily Food Allowance lists on pages 54–69 or make your selection from the menu below.

6.00–7.00 p.m.

Select Carbohydrate for dinner no more than
THREE times per week.

The pattern for dinner is simple.

Remember these
Carbohydrates are
additional to your
daily allowance.

1 Protein	1 Fat	Unlimited Vegetables and salad (not potato, corn, kumara, taro, yams)	1 to 2 Carbohydrates 3 times a week only

On Carbohydrate-free nights, choose ONE Protein serving and grill, bake or stir-fry.

Use ONE Fat serving to cook with or to use as a salad dressing.

Fill your plate to the brim with heaps of vegetables – remember not to include any Carbohydrate vegetables.

On the Carbohydrate nights follow the same procedure but add ONE to TWO Carbohydrates of your choice. Not difficult is it?

Recipes using a Carbohydrate serving have been marked with ⎡C⎤ in the right-hand corner for quick reference. As examples I have listed a selection of Carbohydrate dinner recipes below.

Baked Shrimp, Feta and Lime Parcels (refer page 175)

Verde Fettucine with Ham, Peas and Mascarpone (refer page 192)

Grilled Lamb Burger with Mediterranean Vegetables (refer page 186)

Lemony Orzo with Roast Pumpkin, Red Onion and Feta (refer page 200)

Dessert recipes that use a Carbohydrate have also been identified, for example, *Banana and Date Shortcake* (refer page 229).

When you select one of these dinner or dessert recipes it will become one of your Carbohydrates for that night and you will select only ONE other Carbohydrate to eat with your evening meal.

The chart below will show you ways of turning your Carbohydrate-free dinners into Carbohydrate meals.

Carbohydrate-free Meals	On Carbohydrate nights add in . . .
Hot off the Grill Cracked Peppered Steak, 100 grams, served with mushrooms, tomatoes, steamed green beans	200 grams potatoes
French Lamb Cutlets with Herb Crust (refer page 184) served with peas, carrots, broccoli	1 cup mashed potato
In the Wok *Chicken, Cashew and Pineapple Stir-fry* (refer page 166) *Marinated Teriyaki Lamb with Baby Beans* (refer page 185) *Marmalade and Ginger Pork* (refer page 188)	1 cup cooked rice 100 grams noodles 200 grams kumara
Sauté *Spiced fish with Coconut Lime Raita* (refer page 176) served with steamed broccoli on the side	1 cup cooked rice
Roast Dinner *Roasted Chicken* (refer page 173) served with pumpkin, steamed beans, cauliflower	100 grams potato and 100 grams kumara, roasted
Vegetarian *Falafel with Minted Yoghurt Dressing* (refer page 198)	1 medium pita pocket

Dinner can be served with tea or coffee.

After dinner snack/dessert

Sometimes we just need a little sweet treat to finish off our day. Each day you have the following allowances available to you.

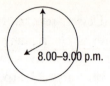

8.00–9.00 p.m.

There are three ways that you can utilise these allowances to create a snack, a supper or an amazing dessert.

1 Fruit	1–2 Milk/Yoghurt	Bits on the Side and Sheer Indulgence (if not used)

1. Basic snack or supper

You may choose to eat a piece of fruit after your dinner or later in the night enjoy ¹/₄ cup yoghurt as a supper **or** you may choose to put the two together for a dessert of fruit and yoghurt.

2. Add in A Bit on the Side or a Sheer Indulgence

On the days you have not used your Bit on the Side, you could create one of these tasty treats.

Caramelised Fruit	1 fruit serving, e.g. 2 fresh apricots cut in half with the stones removed, sprinkled with 2 teaspoons sugar, grilled until sugar is caramelised and served with a ¹/₄ cup yoghurt.
Grilled Sugared Cinnamon Peaches with Whipped Cream and Sliced Almond	(refer page 223)
Fruit Smoothie	¹/₂ cup milk, 1 small banana, 1 teaspoon honey, pinch of cinnamon and 2 ice cubes whipped together until thick and frothy.

3. Add a Carbohydrate   C

On the nights that you have chosen to use your extra Carbohydrate, you could either save one of your Carbohydrate servings from during the day or use one instead of two for dinner. This enables you to create delicious recipes using filo pastry or crumble toppings on your fruit, for example:

Banana Split (refer page 77)

Mixed Berries and Apple Almond Crumble (refer page 225).

Planning either a dessert or a supper can ensure that we do not visit the pantry late at night. I have found it effective to allocate the times I will have my after-dinner snack so that I can look forward to that time rather than sitting there fighting the temptation for a sweet nibble.

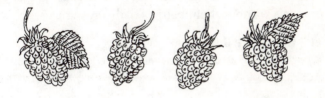

Food Planners
Four weeks of planned meals

Week 1

Monday

Monday, for all of us, seems to be the perfect day to begin our new eating regime. Planning ahead for the week allows us to shop, prepare and then enjoy our meals without them being a daily pressure.

Breakfast – Eat before 9.00 a.m.

You can choose any breakfast that you wish from choices on pages 55 and 71, but I suggest that for the first week you begin with a quick and simple choice, such as fruit and cereal.

$3/4$ cup cornflakes
1 Fruit serving of your choice e.g. 2 kiwifruit
$1/2$ cup milk or $1/4$ cup yoghurt
Tea/Coffee

Morning Tea 10.00 a.m.

If you ate breakfast between 6.00 and 7.00 a.m. you may use
1 Fruit serving of your choice and $1/4$ cup yoghurt
or
If you ate breakfast between 7.00 and 8.30 a.m. you may use
1 Fruit serving of your choice
Tea/Coffee

Lunch 12.00–1.00 p.m.

Remember this is when we metabolise our food most efficiently, so never skimp on your lunch. Make sure you always use the allowances allotted to this time zone. When we talk sandwiches – we want them to be BIG.

BLAT – Bacon, Lettuce and Tomato Sandwich (refer page 73)
Tea/Coffee

Early afternoon snack 2.00 p.m.

1 Fruit serving of your choice

Late afternoon snack 3.30–4.00 p.m.

1 slice wholemeal bread, toasted, spread with 1 teaspoon butter and 2 teaspoons jam
Tea/Coffee

Dinner 6.00–7.00 p.m. | Carbohydrate-free Night |

French Lamb Cutlets with Herb Crust and Creamy Minted Sauce (refer page 184) served with peas, carrots and cauliflower
Tea/Coffee

Supper 8.00–9.00 p.m.

1 Fruit serving of your choice
Tea/Coffee

Tuesday

I hope you enjoyed the menu yesterday and that you are convinced that you are definitely not going to be hungry.

Breakfast – Eat before 9.00 a.m.

$^3/_4$ cup cornflakes
1 Fruit serving of your choice e.g. 1 small banana
$^1/_2$ cup milk or $^1/_4$ cup yoghurt
Tea/Coffee

Morning tea 10.00 a.m.

Continue as you did yesterday and make your choice based on the time you ate breakfast.

Early breakfast – choose 1 Fruit serving and $^1/_4$ cup yoghurt

or

Later breakfast – choose 1 Fruit serving of your choice
Tea/Coffee

Lunch 12.00–1.00 p.m.

We are going to enjoy a luxury week and will be using smoked salmon and dill again for dinner on Wednesday, so when buying your 100 grams smoked salmon for lunch today, buy an extra 50 grams per person ready for the dinner.

Smoked Salmon and Cream Cheese Sandwich
Spead 2 slices of grainy sandwich bread with 1 teaspoon cream cheese and top with 100 grams smoked salmon, thin cucumber slices, pinch of salt, ground black pepper and chopped dill or parsley.
Tea/Coffee

Early afternoon snack 2.00 p.m.

Peckish? How about a piece of fruit to tide you over?

1 serving of seasonal Fruit

Late afternoon snack 3.30–4.00 p.m.
2 Ryvitas spread with 1 tablespoon avocado and topped with slices of tomato, alfalfa sprouts, salt and ground black pepper
Tea/Coffee

Dinner 6.00–7.00 p.m. | Carbohydrate-free Night |
Chicken, Cashew and Pineapple Stir-fry (refer page 166) served with steamed green beans and cauliflower
Tea/Coffee

Supper 8.00–9.00 p.m.
No fruit for supper tonight as we have used the fruit allowance at dinner.
Enjoy a serving of fruity yoghurt instead.
Tea/Coffee

Wednesday

Breakfast – Eat before 9.00 a.m.
You can change the cereal if you wish. I didn't want you to have to buy a different packet of a cereal for each day.
$^3/_4$ cup cornflakes
1 Fruit serving of your choice
$^1/_2$ cup Trim milk or $^1/_4$ cup yoghurt
Tea/Coffee

Morning tea 10.00 a.m.
1 fruit serving and $^1/_4$ cup yoghurt
or
1 Fruit serving of your choice
Tea/Coffee

Lunch 12.00–1.00 p.m.
Two open sandwiches always seem twice as much as one ordinary sandwich. I know some of you won't like cottage cheese – you can substitute feta cheese or chicken if you want to.

Cottage Cheese and Seed Mustard Open Sandwiches on Toast
Toast 2 slices of wholemeal bread and spread with seed mustard. Layer each slice with lettuce, aduki beans, alfalfa sprouts and tomato and cucumber chunks. Top with 125 grams cottage cheese and sprinkle with 1 teaspoon toasted sesame seeds.
Tea/Coffee

Early afternoon tea 2.00 p.m.

Dried fruits can be handy here. If you're on the run they are easy to eat without any mess.

    1 Fruit serving of your choice, e.g. 4 dried apricot halves

Late afternoon tea 3.30–4.00 p.m.

My slice of toast is a little highlight in my afternoon – always use the best jam – not diet.

    1 slice wholemeal bread, toasted and spread with 1 teaspoon butter and 2 teaspoons jam
    Tea/Coffee

Dinner 6.00–7.00 p.m. $\boxed{\text{C}}$ This is the symbol for Carbohydrate Nights

    Smoked Salmon, Bacon and Dill Fettucine (refer page 179) served with steamed broccoli on the side and fresh tomato chunks on top of the fettucine
    Tea/Coffee

Supper 8.00–9.00 p.m.

We will be using melon again on Friday night – save some for then.

    1 cup melon cubes and 1/4 cup yoghurt
    Tea/Coffee

Thursday

Breakfast – Eat before 9.00 a.m.

If you are ready for a change of menu for breakfast feel free to select from the list.

    3/4 cup cornflakes
    1 Fruit serving of your choice
    1/2 cup Trim milk or 1/4 cup yoghurt
    Tea/Coffee

Morning tea 10.00 a.m.

Remember you are selecting your snack here based on your breakfast time.

    1 Fruit serving of your choice and 1/4 cup youghurt
or
    1 Fruit serving
    Tea/Coffee

Lunch 12.00–1.00 p.m.
Be creative with your sandwich fillings. Make a layered sandwich with lettuce top and bottom – it looks wonderful when cut diagonally.
> *Curried Egg Sandwich* (refer page 73)
> Tea/Coffee

Early afternoon snack 2.00 p.m.
> 1 Fruit serving of your choice

Late afternoon snack 3.30–4.00 p.m.
I make up a little jar of mixed seeds, e.g. pumpkin, sesame and sunflower, to sprinkle on my crackers, cereals and salads. Try it here with this snack.
> 2 Ryvita crackers spread with 1 teaspoon butter, vegemite and sprinkled with 2 teaspoons mixed seeds
> Tea/Coffee

Dinner 6.00–7.00 p.m. | Carbohydrate-free Night |
This might be a Carbohydrate-free night, but we can still enjoy a piece of baked pumpkin.
> *Glazed Marinated Pork Chop* (refer page 189) served with baked pumpkin, steamed broccoli and courgettes

Dessert
A little treat to finish off our meal.

> *Honeyed Orange*
> Peel and thinly slice 1 orange. Place in small ovenproof dish and drizzle with 2 teaspoons liquid honey. Grill until hot. Serve swirled with $1/4$ cup yoghurt.
> Tea/Coffee

Friday
Do you realise that by keeping your breakfasts simple you are already successful on one third of your weekly meals?

Breakfast – Eat before 9.00 a.m.
> $3/4$ cup cornflakes
> 1 Fruit serving of your choice
> $1/2$ cup Trim milk or $1/4$ cup yoghurt
> Tea/Coffee

Morning tea 10.00 a.m.
1 Fruit serving and ¼ cup yoghurt
or
1 Fruit serving
Tea/Coffee

Lunch 12.00–1.00 p.m.
Use up the other half of your cottage cheese for lunch today.

Toasted Layered Cottage Cheese Salad Pockets
Pita pockets when lightly toasted become a crisp warm shell. I have layered
these pockets because I enjoy biting through the different textures.
Lightly toast 2 small pita pockets. Line with lettuce leaves. Combine tomato
chunks, 2 sliced gherkins, chopped parsley, 1 teaspoon mayonnaise,
2 tablespoons natural yoghurt, salt and ground black pepper. Use 125 grams
cottage cheese. Spoon ¼ cottage cheese into each pocket, top with
¼ tomato mixture and repeat to use the remaining ingredients.
Tea/Coffee

Early afternoon tea snack 2.00 p.m.
1 Fruit serving of your choice

Late afternoon tea snack 3.30–4.00 p.m.
I hope you are enjoying this toast. If you prefer, you could use crackers and
chutney.
1 slice wholemeal bread, toasted, spread with 1 teaspoon butter and
1 teaspoon marmalade or jam
Tea/Coffee

Dinner 6.00–7.00 p.m. $\boxed{\text{C}}$
Select your Carbohydrate Nights to suit the recipe. This is a perfect combination.
Spiced Fish Topped with Coconut Lime Raita (refer page 176) served with
1 cup cooked rice and steamed broccoli
Tea/Coffee

Supper 8.00–9.00 p.m.
1 cup melon cubes and ¼ cup yoghurt
Tea/Coffee

Saturday

Breakfast

Need a change from your fruit and cereal? You probably don't have to rush off to work today and may have more time to enjoy a cooked breakfast. If you wish, continue with your fruit and cereal.

Egg on Toast
1 slice wholemeal bread, toasted, spread with 1 teaspoon butter, topped with 1 poached egg and sprinkled with a pinch of salt and cayenne pepper. Garnish with chopped parsley.
Tea/Coffee

Morning tea 10.00 a.m.

I hope you are into the swing of these morning-tea snacks.
   1 Fruit serving and ¼ cup yoghurt
or
   1 Fruit serving
   Tea/Coffee

Lunch 12.00–1.00 p.m.

Baked potatoes with different toppings are a wonderful quick stand-by for weekend lunches. Try them topped with baked beans or tuna and mayonnaise, but the bacon and coleslaw is my favourite.
Layered Hot Baked Potatoes for Lunch (refer page 213)
   Tea/Coffee

Combined afternoon snacks 3.00 p.m.

Get baking – because today we are combining our snacks so that we can enjoy this delicious cake for afternoon tea. Freeze the other servings to use next week.
   1 serving of *Ginger-Beer Cake* (refer page 232)
   Tea/Coffee

Dinner 6.00–7.00 p.m. | Carbohydrate-free Night |

If you haven't used all your Sheer Indulgences you might enjoy a glass of wine with your steak tonight.

Grilled Cracked Pepper Steak
Press cracked peppercorns into a 120 grams of scotch fillet steak. Grill on high to your personal preference. Serve with grilled tomatoes, and use 1 teaspoon oil to stir-fry a medley of spring onion, garlic, broccoli florets and mushrooms. Season with soy sauce if you wish.

Dessert
We are using more cream tomorrow night – save some.

Peaches and Cream
$1/2$ cup canned peaches, drained, topped with 3 tablespoons whipped cream
Tea/Coffee

Sunday

Breakfast
I hope that this is music to your ears – for breakfast today it is time for a new cereal and I have named it.
A Symphony of Grains, Seeds and Fruits (refer page 154)
$1/2$ cup milk or $1/4$ cup yoghurt
Tea/Coffee

Morning tea 10.00 a.m.
1 Fruit serving and $1/4$ cup yoghurt
or
1 Fruit serving
Tea/Coffee

Lunch 12.00–1.00 p.m.
This is my at-home café meal. Add grilled tomatoes and mushrooms if you want to bulk it up.

French Toast topped with Grilled Bacon and Maple Syrup
Beat together 1 egg with 2 tablespoons Trim milk, salt and ground black pepper. Dip 2 slices wholemeal bread in mixture to coat. Melt 1 teaspoon butter in a non-stick pan and fry bread until golden on both sides. Grill 1 slice bacon and serve on top of French toast. Drizzle with 1 teaspoon maple syrup.
Tea/Coffee

Combined afternoon tea 3.00 p.m.
The treats go on. You will be pleased that you baked this cake yesterday.
1 serving *Ginger-Beer Cake*
Tea/Coffee

Dinner 6.00–7.00 p.m. [C]

Tonight we are going to have a traditional roast dinner. This is always one of my Carbohydrate nights. Save 100 grams of chicken breast for lunch tomorrow. Then take advantage of the oven being on and bake a delicious dessert.

Roast Chicken Dinner with the Works
Serve 100 grams roast chicken with 120 grams roast potato, 1/2 cup sweetcorn, mashed carrot, parsnip and Brussels sprouts (I love Brussels sprouts but, if you prefer, have beans or peas).

Dessert

Baked Apple Stuffed with Crystallized Ginger (refer page 227) served with 3 tablespoons freshly whipped cream
Tea/Coffee

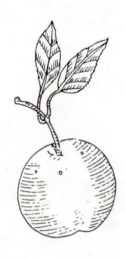

Week 2

Monday

You should be starting to get the hang of this by now – I bet you can't wait for another week to begin. Here goes.

Breakfast
A Symphony of Grains, Seeds and Fruits (refer page 154)
$^1/_2$ cup Trim milk or $^1/_4$ cup yoghurt
Tea/Coffee

Morning tea 10.00 a.m.
Vary your fruit choices. Pick seasonal fruits.
    1 Fruit serving of your choice and $^1/_4$ cup yoghurt
or
    1 Fruit serving
    Tea/Coffee

Lunch 12.00–1.00 p.m.
We are using the chicken you saved from last night's roast dinner. I thought we would use the medium pita pockets this week – they hold heaps of filling and always look generous.
    Chicken Caesar Salad Pocket (refer page 74)
    Tea/Coffee

Early afternoon snack 2.00 p.m.
Use only $^1/_2$ Fruit serving as dessert tonight uses $1^1/_2$ Fruits.
    1 kiwifruit

Late afternoon snack 3.30–4.00 p.m.
    1 slice wholemeal bread, toasted, and spread with 1 teaspoon peanut butter
    Tea/Coffee

Dinner 6.00–7.00 p.m. | Carbohydrate-free Night |
Just as a suggestion, boil sausages before grilling them to remove the excess fat.

    Sausages off the Grill
    2 small sausages, grilled and served with *Spiced Cabbage Stir-fry* (refer page 218)

Dessert

Some days a piece of fruit just doesn't do it for me – but a little dessert does.

Arabian Fruit Salad
Chop and mix together 2 dates, 1 dried fig, 2 dried apricots. Fold in ¼ cup apricot yoghurt.
Tea/Coffee

Tuesday

Breakfast

I hope you are enjoying this week's cereal, but if you want to return to your cornflakes or another choice please do so.
A Symphony of Grains, Seeds and Fruit
½ cup Trim milk or ¼ cup yoghurt
Tea/Coffee

Morning tea 10.00 a.m.

Try different flavoured yoghurts. There are some interesting combinations out there. I recently found rhubarb and rosehip, and a banana and Spirulina.
1 Fruit serving and ¼ cup yoghurt
or
1 Fruit serving
Tea/Coffee

Lunch 12.00–1.00 p.m.

Greek Style Cottage Cheese Open Faced Sandwich
Spread 2 slices of grainy bread with 1 tablespoon avocado. Top each slice of bread with lettuce leaves, 125 grams cottage cheese, chives, cubes of tomato and cucumber and slices of red/green pepper, and sprinkle with 1 teaspoon toasted sesame seeds.
Tea/Coffee

Combined afternoon tea snack

1 serving *Ginger-Beer Cake* (refer page 232)
Tea/Coffee

Dinner 6.00–7.00 p.m. [C]

Marinated Teriyaki Lamb Stir-fry with Baby Beans (refer page 185) served with 1 cup of Hokkien noodles

Dessert

$^1/_2$ cup canned peaches, drained, served with $^1/_4$ cup yoghurt
Tea/Coffee

Wednesday

Breakfast

Yoghurt, if you like it, makes a great change from the milk – sort of sticks to the cereal and makes crunchy clusters – true!
A Symphony of Grains, Seeds and Fruit
$^1/_2$ cup milk or $^1/_4$ cup yoghurt
Tea/Coffee

Morning tea 10.00 a.m.

1 Fruit serving and $^1/_4$ cup yoghurt
or
1 Fruit serving
Tea/Coffee

Lunch 12.00–1.00 p.m.

Bacon and Egg Salad Sandwich
Use 2 slices wholemeal bread and spread them with 1 teaspoon butter. Top with lettuce leaves, snowpeas, 1 rasher grilled bacon, 1 hard-boiled egg, sliced, salt and pepper.
Tea/Coffee

Early afternoon tea snack 2.00 p.m.

1 Fruit serving of your choice

Late afternoon tea snack 3.30–4.00 p.m.

2 crackers spread with 1 tablespoon chutney
Tea/Coffee

Dinner 6.00–7.00 p.m. $\boxed{\text{C}}$

Fish and Chips
Herb and Lemon Fish Parcels served with *Seasoned Potato Chips* (refer page 182)
Tea/Coffee

Supper 8.00–9.00 p.m.

1 cup melon, served with $^1/_4$ cup yoghurt or 1 Fruit serving of your choice
Tea/Coffee

Thursday

Who would want to skip breakfast when you have this delicious cereal mix to look forward to?

Breakfast – Eat before 9.00 a.m.
A Symphony of Grains, Seeds and Fruit
1/2 cup milk or 1/4 cup yoghurt
Tea/Coffee

Morning tea 10.00 a.m.
1 Fruit serving of your choice with 1/4 cup yoghurt
or
1 Fruit serving of your choice
Tea/Coffee

Lunch 12.00–1.00 p.m.
I also enjoy this pâté served on top of a hot baked potato – you might like to try it that way for a change.
Chunky Salmon Pâté (refer page 174) served with 2 slices of toast, spread with 1 teaspoon butter and cut into fingers
Tea/Coffee

Early afternoon tea snack 2.00 p.m.
1 Fruit serving of your choice

Late afternoon snack 3.30–4.00 p.m.
2 crackers spread with 1 tablespoon avocado and topped with tomato slices, salt, ground black pepper and alfalfa sprouts
Tea/Coffee

Dinner 6.00–7.00 p.m.   Carbohydrate-free Night
Chicken Thighs with a Coat of Many Spices (refer page 167) served with steamed beans, cauliflower and carrots

Dessert
1/2 cup stewed apple served with 1/4 cup custard or yoghurt
Tea/Coffee

Friday

Breakfast
Breakfast may seem repetitive but the idea is to get you into a routine.
Find your own rut.
> *A Symphony of Grains, Seeds and Fruit*
> $1/2$ cup milk or $1/4$ cup yoghurt
> Tea/Coffee

Morning tea 10.00 a.m.
> 1 Fruit serving of your choice and $1/4$ cup yoghurt

or
> 1 Fruit serving of your choice
> Tea/Coffee

Lunch 12.00–1.00 p.m.
> *A Many Bean Salad with Toasted Pita Pockets* (refer page 203)
> Tea/Coffee

Early afternoon 2.00 p.m.
> 1 Fruit serving of your choice

Late afternoon snack 3.30–4.00 p.m.
> 1 crumpet, toasted, spread with 1 teaspoon butter and Vegemite/Marmite
> Tea/Coffee

Dinner 6.00–7.00 p.m. | Carbohydrate-free Night |
> *Marmalade and Ginger Pork Stir-fry* (refer page 188) served with broccoli

Dessert
> $1/2$ cup canned peaches with $1/4$ cup yoghurt
> Tea/Coffee

Saturday

Breakfast
I hope that you are beginning to love this way of eating as much as I do. However, in case you can't face another cereal breakfast, we have a sweet fruit compote today
> *Gingered Fruit Compote* (refer page 158) served with $1/4$ cup yoghurt
> Tea/Coffee

Morning tea 10.00 a.m.

1 Fruit serving with ¼ cup yoghurt

or

1 Fruit serving of your choice
Tea/Coffee

Lunch 12.00–1.00 p.m.

Potato Fritters for Lunch with a Lemon Sweet Chilli Sauce (refer page 215)
Tea/Coffee

Early afternoon snack 2.00 p.m.

1 Fruit serving of your choice

Late afternoon snack 3.30–4.00 p.m.

2 Ryvitas spread with 1 tablespoon avocado and topped with sliced tomatoes, black pepper and alfalfa.
Tea/Coffee

Dinner 6.00–7.00 p.m. | Carbohydrate-free Night |

Let's be wild here and enjoy the Sheer Indulgence of a glass of wine.

Spiced Fillet of Beef Salad with Char-grilled Red Pepper Vinaigrette (refer page 159)

Dessert

½ cup canned apricots served with ¼ cup yoghurt
Tea/Coffee

Sunday

Breakfast

You can soak the oats the night before or make it fresh in the morning – either way it is delicious.

Bircher Muesli (refer page 157)
Tea/Coffee

Morning tea 10.00 a.m.

Remember how this works – if you get up late and eat later than 9 a.m. you only have a cup of tea or coffee. Early risers get the following choices.

1 Fruit serving and ¼ cup yoghurt

or

1 Fruit serving
Tea/Coffee

Lunch 12.00–1.00 p.m.
Herbed Scrambled Eggs (refer page 74)
Tea/Coffee

Early afternoon tea 2.00 p.m.
Just a half Fruit serving again today – enjoy the muffin later.
1 kiwifruit

Late afternoon tea snack 3.30–4.00 p.m.
Let's get baking again and stock up for next week.
1 *Blueberry Muffin* (refer page 231)
Tea/Coffee

Dinner 6.00–7.00 p.m. | Carbohydrate-free Night |
Finish the week off with a roast of lamb seasoned with rosemary. A roast dinner is my favourite meal, especially when served with roast potato and kumara. Keep some cold meat for tomorrow and make a delicious sandwich with chutney.

The Big Kiwi Roast Leg-of-Lamb Dinner
Serve 100 grams cooked roast lamb with 100 grams roast potato and 100 grams kumara, small wedge pumpkin, and steamed green beans. Drizzle with mint sauce.

Dessert
Poached Pear in a Ginger Vanilla Sugar Syrup
Peel pear, remove core and cut in quarters. In a small pot gently heat 1/2 cup water, 2 teaspoons Vanilla Sugar (refer page 233) and 1 slice root ginger. Add pears and simmer for 8 minutes until pear is softened and syrup has thickened. Serve hot or cold, swirled with 1/4 cup yoghurt.
Tea/Coffee

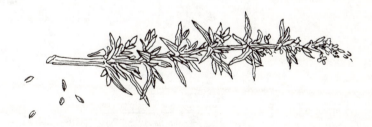

Week 3

Monday

Breakfast – Eat before 9.00 a.m.
Once you have mixed up your own cereal combinations you won't want to buy the commercial range – they taste so much better and the fruits are softer.
A Bit of a Mix-up (refer page 156)
serve with ¼ cup yoghurt
Tea/Coffee

Morning tea 10.00 a.m.
1 Fruit serving of your choice and ¼ cup yoghurt
or
1 Fruit serving of your choice
Tea/Coffee

Lunch 12.00–1.00 p.m.
The best thing about serving a roast on Sunday night is that I always have cold meat for my lunch on Monday.

Lamb and Chutney Sandwich
Spread 2 slices of wholemeal bread with 1 teaspoon butter. Layer one slice of bread with lettuce leaf, tomato slices, sprouts, 100 grams thinly sliced lamb, salt and pepper. Top with ½ tablespoon fruit chutney, lettuce leaf and bread.
Tea/Coffee

Early afternoon snack 2.00 p.m.
½ fruit serving of your choice, e.g. 1 kiwifruit, or 2 dried apricot halves

Late afternoon snack 3.30–4.00 p.m.
1 *Blueberry Muffin*
Tea/Coffee

Dinner 6.00–7.00 p.m.   Carbohydrate-free Night
Curried Sausages with Mashed Carrots and Parsnips on the Side
Boil and skin 2 medium sausages then cut into chunks. Heat a large pot, add a little water and sauté ½ onion until tender. Add 1 teaspoon medium curry powder and cook for 2 minutes. Add 1 carrot, 1 stick celery, sausages, ½ cup water and squeeze lemon juice. Cover and simmer for 15 minutes. Add ¼ cup frozen peas then reduce heat. Thicken with 1 teaspoon cornflour

mixed to a paste with a little water and season with salt and ground black pepper. Serve with 1 cup mashed carrots and parsnip.
Tea/Coffee

Supper 8.00–9.00 p.m.
1 Fruit serving of your choice and $^1/_4$ cup yoghurt
Tea/Coffee

Tuesday

Breakfast – Eat before 9.00 a.m.
A Bit of a Mix-up (refer page 156)
serve with $^1/_4$ cup yoghurt
Tea/Coffee

Morning tea 10.00 a.m.
Early breakfast – choose 1 Fruit serving and $^1/_4$ cup yoghurt
or
1 Fruit serving of your choice
Tea/Coffee

Lunch 12.00–1.00 p.m.
Tuna and Mayonnaise Pita Pocket
Split 1 medium pita pocket and line with lettuce leaves. Mix together 100 grams tuna, 1 teaspoon mayonnaise, pinch of salt and ground black pepper. Spoon tuna into pocket and top with tomato and cucumber chunks.
Tea/Coffee

Early afternoon snack 2.00 p.m.
Only $^1/_2$ Fruit serving here so we can have a fruit salad for dessert. Use 1 plum, kiwifruit, or dried fruit.
$^1/_2$ Fruit serving of your choice

Late afternoon snack 3.30–4.00 p.m.
Cinnamon Toast (refer page 233)
Tea/Coffee

Dinner 6.00–7.00 p.m. | Carbohydrate-free Night |
Coconut Chicken with a Touch of Spice (refer page 170) served with a mixture of steamed vegetables – broccoli, carrots and cauliflower.

Dessert
Mini Fruit Salad
¹/₂ orange, ¹/₂ banana, 1 kiwifruit cut into chunks and topped with ¹/₄ cup yoghurt
Tea/Coffee

Wednesday

Breakfast
A Bit of a Mix-up
serve with ¹/₄ cup yoghurt
Tea/Coffee

Morning tea 10.00 a.m.
1 Fruit serving and ¹/₄ cup yoghurt
or
1 Fruit serving of your choice
Tea/Coffee

Lunch 12.00–1.00 p.m.
I find eggs so convenient for my lunches, and when mashed hot with curry powder and mixed beans sprouts they're crunchy and filling. Look for interesting grainy breads to create variety in your lunch.
Curried Egg Sandwich (refer page 73)
Tea/Coffee

Early afternoon tea 2.00 p.m.
As we are using our Blueberry Muffins this week it means this snack is still half a Fruit serving.
¹/₂ Fruit serving of your choice

Late afternoon tea 3.30–4.00 p.m.
1 *Blueberry Muffin*
Tea/Coffee

Dinner 6.00–7.00 p.m.   C
Grilled Lamb Burger with Mediterranean Vegetables (refer page 186)
Tea/Coffee

Supper 8.00–9.00 p.m.
1 fruit serving of your choice and $1/4$ cup yoghurt
Tea/Coffee

Thursday

Breakfast – Eat before 9.00 a.m.
Remember that you can always change the cereal for another choice off your Breakfast Package list – the main thing is to not skip breakfast.
A Bit of a Mix-up
serve with $1/4$ cup yoghurt
Tea/Coffee

Morning tea 10.00 a.m.
1 Fruit serving of your choice and $1/4$ cup yoghurt
or
1 Fruit serving
Tea/Coffee

Lunch 12.00–1.00 p.m.
Crispy mixed sprouts are a must in the fridge – they transform any sandwich or stir-fry with their nutty texture.

Crispy Mixed Bean Sprouts and Cottage Cheese Pockets
Lightly toast 2 small pita pockets. Line with lettuce leaves and fill with 125 grams cottage cheese mixed with 1 teaspoon pesto and mixed bean sprouts.
Tea/Coffee

Early afternoon snack 2.00 p.m.
1 Fruit serving of your choice

Late afternoon snack 3.30–4.00 p.m.
2 Ryvita crackers spread with 1 tablespoon avocado, alfalfa, tomato slices and seasoned with a pinch of salt and lots of ground black pepper.
Tea/Coffee

Dinner 6.00–7.00 p.m. | Carbohydrate-free Night |

Honey Lemon Chicken Stir-fry
Heat 1 teaspoon oil in non-stick pan and sauté 120 grams chicken breast/ thighs cut into small chunks with garlic and grated root ginger until well cooked. Add chopped celery, carrot strips and cook until tender. Add finely shredded cabbage and spring onion – cook 2 minutes. Add 1 tablespoon

soy sauce, 1 teaspoon honey, 1 teaspoon lemon juice, 1/2 teaspoon chicken
stock and stir until chicken and vegetables are well coated.
Tea/Coffee

Supper 8.00–9.00 p.m.
1 fruit serving of your choice with 1/4 cup yoghurt
Tea/Coffee

Friday
Friday is always my favourite day because I end my busy week and look
forward to some time at home. Take a deep breath and launch into the
day with the thought that the weekend is looming.

Breakfast
A Bit of a Mix-Up
serve with 1/4 cup yoghurt
Tea/Coffee

Morning tea 10.00 a.m.
1 Fruit serving and 1/4 cup yoghurt
or
1 Fruit serving
Tea/Coffee

Lunch 12.00–1.00 p.m.
I could eat this sandwich every day – it's my favourite!

Blat
Spread 2 slices wholemeal bread with 1 tablespoon avocado. Fill with lettuce,
2 rashers grilled bacon, tomato slices, salt and ground black pepper.
Tea/Coffee

Early afternoon snack 2.00 p.m.
1/2 Fruit serving of your choice

Late afternoon snack 3.30–4.00 p.m.
Don't knock this until you try it.
1 slice wholemeal bread, toasted and spread with 1 teaspoon peanut butter
and 1/2 banana, mashed
Tea/Coffee

Dinner 6.00–7.00 p.m. | Carbohydrate-free Night |

Grilled Fish with tomato pesto
Spread 140 grams fish fillet with 1 teaspoon tomato pesto and ground black pepper. Grill for 4 minutes on each side. Serve with grilled slices of courgette, steamed baby spinach leaves and carrots.

Dessert
1/4 cup pineapple pieces served with 1/4 cup yoghurt
Tea/Coffee

Saturday

Breakfast
Revisit the Breakfast Package List on your food plan and see if there is anything you would like for a change. If not, try my selection.
Bircher Muesli (refer page 157)
Tea/Coffee

Morning tea 10.00 a.m.
1 Fruit serving and 1/4 cup yoghurt
or
1 Fruit serving
Tea/Coffee

Lunch 12.00–1.00 p.m.
Herbed Soufflé Omelet (refer page 205) served with triangles of wholemeal toast (2 slices)
Tea/Coffee

Early afternoon 2.00 p.m.
1/2 Fruit serving of your choice

Late afternoon 3.30–4.00 p.m.
10 thin rice wafers served with dip of your choice (refer page 222)
Tea/Coffee

Dinner 6.00–7.00 p.m. C
Roasted Pork Fillet Mignon with Button Mushroom Sauce (refer page 190) served with 120 grams baked jacket kumara and vegetables of your choice.

Dessert
Use one Sheer Indulgence for your cream – it's better than yoghurt.

> *Banana and Date Shortcake* (refer page 229)
> served hot with 3 tablespoons whipped cream
> Tea/Coffee

Sunday
This is the last day of your planners. I hope you have enjoyed the meals that I have selected for you. From here you can repeat the last three weeks or begin to create your own menus using the recipes that follow plus your own favourites.

Breakfast
We are going to finish this week with a wonderful treat for breakfast.
> *Breakfast Pancakes with Lemon Honey* (refer page 155)
> Tea/Coffee

Morning tea 10.00 a.m.
> 1 Fruit serving and ¼ cup yoghurt

or

> 1 Fruit serving
> Tea/Coffee

Lunch 12.00–1.00 p.m.
> *Chunky Salmon Pâté* (refer page 174) served with 4 Ryvita crackers and chunks of tomato on the side
> Tea/Coffee

Combined afternoon tea 3.00 p.m.
> *Banana and Date Shortcake*
> Tea/Coffee

Dinner 6.00–7.00 p.m. C
This is a roasted chicken with a yoghurt and spice coating – really superb. Try a squeeze of lemon juice over your broccoli and carrots with lots of ground black pepper.
> *More than a Roasted Chicken* (refer page 173) serve 100 grams roast chicken with 120 grams jacket potato, steamed broccoli, and carrots.

and, YES, a little pudding

Baked Rum Bananas

Peel 1 banana. Cut a square of tin foil and place banana in the middle. Sprinkle with $1/2$ teaspoon soft brown sugar, 1 teaspoon dark rum and orange zest. Roll up and bake in the oven for 10 minutes. (I turn the oven off after cooking the chicken and just pop the parcel in while I am eating dinner.) Serve with $1/4$ cup yoghurt or, if you still have a Sheer Indulgence available, serve with 3 tablespoons whipped cream.

Tea/Coffee

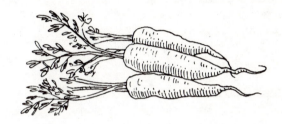

Week on the run

There are some weeks that we just don't have time to think about meals, and that is when we want a no-brain week. I have lots of these!

Monday

Breakfast – Eat before 9.00 a.m.

Use one cereal for the whole week so choose what you have in the cupboard and go for it. Or use as below.

$^3/_4$ cup cornflakes
1 Fruit serving of your choice, e.g. 2 kiwifruit
$^1/_2$ cup milk or $^1/_4$ cup yoghurt
Tea/Coffee

Morning tea 10.00 a.m.

If you ate breakfast between 6.00 and 7.00 a.m. you may use
1 Fruit serving of your choice and $^1/_4$ cup yoghurt
or
If you ate breakfast between 7.00 and 8.30 a.m. you may use
1 Fruit serving of your choice
Tea/Coffee

Lunch 12.00–1.00 p.m.

My lunches are very similar each day. I use my 2 breads, buttered and filled with whatever has survived in the fridge, such as leftovers from my weekend roast.
Sandwich of your choice
Tea/Coffee

Early afternoon snack 2.00 p.m.

1 Fruit serving of your choice

Late afternoon snack 3.30–4.00 p.m.

1 slice wholemeal bread, toasted and spread with 1 teaspoon butter and 2 teaspoons jam
Tea/Coffee

Dinner 6.00–7.00 p.m. | Carbohydrate-free Night |

While fresh vegetables are always my first preference, I do keep a couple of bags of frozen vegetables for those nights I haven't made it to the supermarket.
Grilled lamb chops (2) served with vegetables of your choice
Tea/Coffee

Supper 8.00–9.00 p.m.
1 Fruit serving of your choice and $1/4$ cup yoghurt
Tea/Coffee

Tuesday
Just get that cereal in the bowl and move on into your day.

Breakfast – Eat before 9.00 a.m.
$3/4$ cup cornflakes
1 Fruit serving of your choice, e.g. 1 small banana
$1/2$ cup milk or $1/4$ cup yoghurt
Tea/Coffee

Morning tea 10.00 a.m.
Early breakfast – choose 1 Fruit serving and $1/4$ cup yoghurt
or
Later breakfast – choose 1 Fruit serving of your choice
Tea/Coffee

Lunch 12.00–1.00 p.m.
Curried Egg and Parsley Sandwich
Spread 2 slices of wholemeal bread with 1 teaspoon butter. Fill with 2 eggs, boiled and mashed with $1/2$ teaspoon curry powder, salt and pepper. Add lettuce and lots of sprouts and parsley.
Tea/Coffee

Early afternoon snack 2.00 p.m.
1 serving of seasonal Fruit

Late afternoon snack 3.30–4.00 p.m.
2 Ryvitas spread with 1 tablespoon avocado and topped with slices of tomato, alfalfa sprouts, salt and ground black pepper.
Tea/Coffee

Dinner 6.00–7.00 p.m. C
Cook an extra piece of chicken for tomorrow's lunch – double up the marinade or cook it plain.

Grilled Chicken Breast
Mix together 2 teaspoons Worcestershire sauce, 1 teaspoon seed mustard, $1/2$ teaspoon grated root ginger, $1/2$ teaspoon chilli sauce, 1 crushed garlic clove, salt and ground black pepper. Brush mixture over 120 gram chicken

breast and grill until cooked. Serve with 100 gram potato, ¹/₂ cup sweetcorn and steamed green beans.
Tea/Coffee

Supper 8.00–9.00 p.m.
I throw my fruit under the grill to warm and then drizzle it with yoghurt.
¹/₂ cup canned pears or fruit of your choice topped with ¹/₄ cup yoghurt
Tea/Coffee

Wednesday

Breakfast
Same breakfast so there is no decision to make.
³/₄ cup cornflakes
1 Fruit serving of your choice
¹/₂ cup Trim milk or ¹/₄ cup yoghurt
Tea/Coffee

Morning tea 10.00 a.m.
1 Fruit serving and ¹/₄ cup yoghurt
or
1 Fruit serving of your choice
Tea/Coffee

Lunch 12.00–1.00 p.m.
I find it convenient to buy a bag of mixed salad greens so that I can grab a handful for my sandwich each day without having to do any preparation.
Make a sandwich using 100 grams chicken from last night filled with salad and sprouts of your choice.
Tea/Coffee

Early afternoon tea 2.00 p.m.
1 Fruit serving of your choice

Late afternoon tea 3.30–4.00 p.m.
10 thin rice wafers to eat as you go
Tea/Coffee

Dinner 6.00–7.00 p.m.   Carbohydrate-free Night
Steak and Peppers
Grill 120 grams steak. Serve with sliced red, green and orange peppers, courgettes and cauliflower stir-fried in 1 teaspoon oil.
Tea/Coffee

Supper 8.00–9.00 p.m.
1 Fruit serving of your choice served with $1/4$ cup yoghurt
Tea/Coffee

Thursday

Breakfast
If you are ready for a change of menu for breakfast, feel free to select from the list.
$3/4$ cup cornflakes
1 Fruit serving of your choice
$1/2$ cup Trim milk or $1/4$ cup yoghurt
Tea/Coffee

Morning tea 10.00 a.m.
Remember you are selecting your snack here based on your breakfast time.
1 Fruit serving of your choice and $1/4$ cup yoghurt
or
1 Fruit serving
Tea/Coffee

Lunch 12.00–1.00 p.m.
I enjoy this sandwich with finely chopped spring onion, but only when I am not going to be breathing on anyone!

Salmon and Mayonnaise Sandwich
Spread 2 slices of grainy sandwich bread with 1 teaspoon mayonnaise and top with 100 grams canned salmon, squeeze of lemon and lots of black pepper, thin cucumber slices, alfalfa, pinch of salt and heaps chopped parsley.
Tea/Coffee

Early afternoon snack 2.00 p.m.
1 Fruit serving of your choice

Late afternoon snack 3.30–4.00 p.m.
Of all the snacks, toast is still my favourite.
1 slice toast spread with 1 teaspoon butter and 2 teaspoons marmalade or jam
Tea/Coffee

Dinner 6.00–7.00 p.m. | Carbohydrate-free Night |

Grilled Sausages (2 small) served with grilled tomatoes and mushrooms and steamed beans
Tea/Coffee

Supper 8.00–9.00 p.m.

1 Fruit serving of your choice with $1/4$ cup yoghurt
Tea/Coffee

Friday

Nearly the weekend – hang in there.

Breakfast

$3/4$ cup cornflakes
1 Fruit serving of your choice
$1/2$ cup Trim milk or $1/4$ cup yoghurt
Tea/Coffee

Morning tea 10.00 a.m.

1 Fruit serving and $1/4$ cup yoghurt

or

1 Fruit serving
Tea/Coffee

Lunch 12.00–1.00 p.m.

Big Bacon and Egg Sandwich
Spread 2 slices wholemeal bread with 1 teaspoon butter. Fill with lettuce, thinly sliced tomato, 1 hard-boiled egg, 1 grilled bacon rasher, chopped parsley, salt and ground black pepper.
Tea/Coffee

Early afternoon tea snack 2.00 p.m.

1 Fruit serving of your choice

Late afternoon tea snack 3.30–4.00 p.m.

1 slice wholemeal bread, toasted, spread with 1 teaspoon butter and 2 teaspoons marmalade or jam.

Dinner 6.00–7.00 p.m. | Carbohydrate-free Night |

Fish is my instant meal and this is one I use a lot because it is not only delicious but fast.

Dijon Mustard Grilled Fish
Spread 120 gram fish fillet, skinned and boned, with 1 teaspoon Dijon mustard, ground black pepper, squeeze of lemon juice and 1 teaspoon oil. Grill for 4 minutes on each side. Serve with vegetables of your choice.
Tea/Coffee

Supper 8.00–9.00 p.m.
1/2 cup canned apricots served with 1/4 cup yoghurt
Tea/Coffee

Saturday

If you are like me you probably thought the weekend would never come. Let's give the body a shot of vitamins and minerals with a healthy fresh fruit salad.

Breakfast
Fresh fruit salad using 3 Fruit servings of your choice served with 1/4 cup yoghurt
Tea/Coffee

Morning tea 10.00 a.m.
Another piece of Fruit or you can carry it over to the afternoon.
1 Fruit serving and 1/4 cup yoghurt
or
1 Fruit serving
Tea/Coffee

Lunch 12.00–1.00 p.m.
I find baked beans ideal for a Saturday lunch – hot, quick and filling.

Beans Supreme on Toast
Serve 170 grams hot baked beans on 2 slices toasted bread, covered with alfalfa and mung sprouts. Top with ground black pepper and parsley.
Tea/Coffee

Combined afternoon snack 3.00 p.m.

Let's go domestic briefly and bake a loaf for afternoon tea.
2 slices *Maple Fruit and Nut Loaf* (refer page 234)
Tea/Coffee

Dinner 6.00–7.00 p.m. C

I have split the Carbohydrate between the dinner and the dessert tonight.

Old-fashioned Roast Beef Dinner
Serve 100 grams lean roast beef with 100 grams potato, (roasted in 1 teaspoon oil), 1 wedge pumpkin baked in foil and steamed broccoli.

If you want gravy, here is an instant no-fat one – don't judge it until you try it.
For 1 serving, in a pot place 1 teaspoon Vegemite dissolved in ³/₄ cup boiling water. Stir in 1 teaspoon cornflour mixed with a little water. Simmer until gravy thickens.

Dessert

Apple Crumble
In an ovenproof dish place ¹/₂ cup stewed apple topped with a mix of 4 tablespoons crushed cornflakes and 1 teaspoon each of butter, sugar and ¹/₂ teaspoon of cinnamon. Bake 10–15 minutes at 210°C. Swirl ¹/₄ cup yoghurt on top.
Tea/Coffee

Sunday

We may not be able to change our busy lifestyles, but we can at least change the way that we eat on the run. Often the only changes needed are to the way we shop. Make sure you have all the basic ingredients you need on hand.

Breakfast

There's a slight change of pace this morning.
Poached Egg on Toast (refer page 74)
Tea/Coffee

Morning tea 10.00 a.m.

1 Fruit serving and ¹/₄ cup yoghurt
or
1 Fruit serving
Tea/Coffee

Lunch 12.00–1.00 p.m.

Gourmet Chicken Burger (refer page 169)
Tea/Coffee

Combined afternoon tea 3.00 p.m.

1 serving *Maple Fruit Nut Loaf*
Tea/Coffee

Dinner 6.00–7.00 p.m. | C |

We are using up some of the cold roast beef for dinner tonight. This means one meal we don't have to think about – I like that!

Cold Roast Beef and Irish Mash
100 grams sliced roast beef served with 1 cup mashed potato mixed with spring onion and vegetables of your choice.

Dessert

Ice-cream uses one of your Sheer Indulgences so make sure you haven't used all your allowances. If you have – use yoghurt.

Apricots and Ice-cream
Serve ¹/₂ cup canned apricots with ¹/₄ cup ice-cream
Tea/Coffee

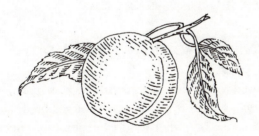

Chapter 4

Hill Grown, Ripened in the Sun

Foods that Might Actually have Some Nutrients in them!

Have you ever paused to consider that eating food is more than just a recreational activity or something to do when you're bored? I know that I am stating the obvious here, but food is a source of energy that is supposed to provide us with the necessary nutrients to not only keep us alive, but to ensure we are healthy. Are the foods we are selecting doing this?

There was a time when our foods were purchased fresh from having touched the earth and seen the sun, but today most of our food is manufactured or processed and travels down the factory conveyor belt encased in an unnatural wrapping of plastic. Food is manufactured at a rate of 3800 calories a day per person, which, if eaten at that rate, explains the increasing rate of obesity. As I observe the food's continued journey down the supermarket conveyor belt I am amazed that it provides any worthwhile nutrition whatsoever, never mind keeping us alive.

At middle-age the nutrients in our foods become of special significance.

All women's experiences of menopause and weight gain are not the same, and it is well documented that women from Japan, Korea and Asia do not have the same negative experiences of menopause, or weight gain, as European women.

Why?

Research suggests it is simply a matter of the differences in the types of food we eat. Japanese women eat foods that contain phytoestrogens, plant hormones that mimic the effect of human estrogen. Research has found that phytoestrogens compete for the same hormone receptor sites as our natural hormones. When our natural estrogen levels are high the phytoestrogen effect is minimised. They effectively plug the gap when needed.

Fortunately, phytoestrogens are naturally occurring substances found in foods such as fruits, vegetables, soy and cereals as well as many of the foods you are probably already eating, and they are readily available. So you can relax. They are not supplements or specialised foods that you are going to have to import from the Himalayas!

To soy or not to soy

Yes, I admit it. I drink soy milk. But I remember, not that many years ago, that if someone joined my class and told me, often in hushed tones, that they didn't drink cows' milk, only soy, I viewed them with suspicion and as strangely 'hippie'. Never say never – times change.

Over the past few years soy products have rocketed into prominence. Our eagerness to use soy has been fuelled by claims in the popular press and health books on its therapeutic advantages. Researchers claim that phytoestrogens inhibit cancer formation in humans, are beneficial for treating osteoporosis, and reduce cholesterol levels. Many of these studies are based on small test samples. However, it was on the basis of research I had read that I made the decision not to drink cows' milk. We are the only mammal to drink another mammal's milk, and many people are lactose intolerant (lactose is a sugar in cows' milk). It is also suggested that the hormones in cows' milk may be recognised by our hormone receptors and cause confusion in our cells. Many other cultures don't drink cows' milk at all and don't seem to suffer any adverse consequences.

Hot flushes are also claimed to be minimised by using soy milk instead of cows' milk. My own experience of using soy milk has been positive. There may be a sound basis for this claim because, as you can see in tables 4.1 and 4.2, soy is rich in phytoestrogens, so it is possible they are supporting our falling estrogen levels.

Whether the benefits are psychological or physical I can't say – the jury is still out on the benefits of soy, but if it works for some of us, don't knock it.

Phytoestrogen (phyto means plant)

There are several categories of phytoestrogens, and I believe it is useful for us to be able to identify foods rich in them and to make an effort to include them in our daily menus.

Table 4.1

Isoflavones	Lignans	Coumestans
chickpeas lentils soy products	cereals seeds • linseed/flaxseed	Sprouted seeds – a concentrated food storage unit rich in nutrients • aduki bean sprouts • alfalfa sprouts • mung bean sprouts

Grind seeds before eating otherwise they will pass through your system unprocessed and without releasing the nutrients.

Phytoestrogens are also found in these foods.

Table 4.2

Cereals	Fruits	Pulses	Soy Products	Herb/Spice	Vegetables
oats rice rye wheat	apples berries cherries citrus plums	kidney beans nuts seeds • pumpkin • sunflower • sesame	miso soy milk soy yoghurt soy sauce tofu	sage parsley cinnamon	broccoli carrots celery garlic peas potatoes

Talk about going a bit nutty

You are right in thinking nuts are high in fat and calories – they can be fattening if you eat too many of them, such as a handful or two with drinks before eating dinner. However, nuts contain phytoestrogens and selenium, both of which are beneficial to us in middle-age (see Tables 4.2 and 4.4). Gram for gram, nuts are nutrient dense so substituting nuts for another protein can be part of a healthy diet.

Feeling a bit 'brittle'?

If you are a woman who is:
- elderly
- Caucasian
- small-framed or
- experiencing early menopause

then you are at risk for osteoporosis, a condition in which there is a loss of bone density, making the bones more vulnerable to fractures. Calcium is an important mineral for bone formation and maintenance.

To reduce your risk of calcium loss and osteoporosis:
- Eat foods daily that are rich in calcium (see Table 4.3)
- Reduce caffeine consumption
- Reduce alcohol consumption
- Get some sunlight
- Exercise regularly – walking and weight-bearing exercise
- Don't overdo the protein – excessive intakes of protein cause an acidic reaction in the body and calcium is leached from the bones to act as a neutraliser. This can create a calcium imbalance, leading to a risk of osteoporosis.

Table 4.3 Calcium-rich foods

Dairy Foods	Non-Dairy Foods
cheese	almonds
cottage cheese	brazils
milk	baked beans
yoghurt	chickpeas
	dried fruit – kiwifruit, raspberries, blackcurrants
	hummus
	parsley
	salmon
	sardines
	seeds – pumpkin/sesame/sunflower
	soy milk/yoghurt
	spinach
	vegetables – silverbeet, spinach, watercress
	tofu
	wholemeal bread

Nature's vitamin cocktail

My doctor once said that taking vitamin supplements was solely for the benefits of the fish at the sewerage ponds. I have only on the rare occasion taken vitamin supplements and prefer to try to ingest my vitamins from fresh food products. There is, of course, the argument that our soils are so depleted of nutrients that we could never eat enough food to meet our daily recommended vitamin intake. I believe we should begin with a balanced daily intake of fresh foods, taking note of foods that contain essential nutrients and then, and only then, top up with supplements if needed. If you do feel you are deficient in a particular nutrient, don't self-diagnose, but rather seek professional help. Wandering down the vitamin aisle at the supermarket and selecting a supplement based on how you feel that day is not an accurate assessment of what you actually need.

Table 4.4   Foods rich in vitamins, minerals and antioxidants

Vitamin A	Vitamin B6	Vitamin B12	Vitamin C	Vitamin E	Zinc	Selenium
carrots	bananas	cheese	berries	avocado	almonds	Brazil nuts
oranges	brown rice	eggs	broccoli	nuts	beans	cabbage
pawpaw	chicken	fish	cauliflower	oily fish	brazil nuts	eggs
peaches	liver	meat	citrus fruit	seeds	cashews	shrimps
pumpkin	tuna	milk/yoghurt	green leafy	vegetable	eggs	tuna
tomatoes		shellfish	vegetables	oil	fish	
(cooked)			kiwifruit	wheatgerm	oysters	
					seeds	

Hormone deficient versus vitamin deficient

When I read the symptoms of vitamin B6 and vitamin B12 deficiency it makes me wonder whether it is the lack of these vitamins that is causing our menopausal symptoms.

Vitamin B6 deficiency:
▶ Anxiety
▶ Depression
▶ Insomnia
▶ Irritability
▶ Vitamin B6 is needed for the production of serotonin – our feel-good neurotransmitter. When our serotonin levels are normal we crave less carbohydrate and sugar and our nervous system is calmed.

Vitamin B12 deficiency:
▶ Difficulty concentrating and remembering
▶ Severe agitation
▶ Manic behaviour.

Oh dear! Sounds all very familiar to me. Time for an egg for breakfast, tuna salad sandwich for lunch, brown-rice chicken risotto for dinner, followed by banana and yoghurt for dessert.

But it's 97% fat-free!

Yes – but that doesn't make it calorie-free.

It is interesting that while the intake of saturated fat has supposedly decreased, obesity has trebled in the past two decades in most Western countries.

The desire to reduce our fat intakes has led to a flood of new products on the market announcing that they are 97% FAT-FREE. The promotion of these products is often deceptive and leaves us with the impression that low fat equates to low calories. This is not always the case.

Each week I meet with people claiming they can't lose weight even though they have been following a virtually no-fat diet. I enjoy asking them what they have been eating. The answer I already know – fat-free muffins, fat-free cakes, fat-free ice-cream, fat-free salad dressing and NO BUTTER for years.

When you compare the labels of fat-free products with their full-fat versions, take note of the calorie value rather than the fat content. You will find that in many cases the calorie content of the fat-free foods is as high or even higher than the other version. That is because sugar and other quickly digested simple carbohydrates are used to replace the fat.

There is only one equation to be considered in weight loss and that is energy in against energy out. It does not help to just substitute carbohydrates, in large amounts, for the fats that have been taken out.

Avoid getting a 'don't-eat-fat' phobia.

We want to lose weight in a normal rather than an artificial environment. Our objective is to make permanent lifestyle changes that will continue well beyond us achieving our desired weight. It is far more enjoyable and helpful for us to learn to use the correct portion of a product rather than thinking we can have more because it is low fat. When we have more of the diet product we end up having the same amount of calories as the product we would prefer.

Aversion therapy

In the United States the use of artificial fats has been approved for use in snack foods. It has been reported that these fats can cause some extremely unpleasant side effects such as 'anal drip' and loose stools. I can assure you that the loose stools do not refer to a wobbly leg on a chair but rather to a form of diarrhoea. Are we really that desperate to eat junk food?

And did you know that chocolate is saturated fat made palatable with sugar?

Okay, enough therapy, time to discuss strategies for eating out.

Surviving the 'Dinner Out'

When trying to lose weight it sometimes feels as if it would be easier to go into isolation rather than having to try to integrate the plan into our social life. Unfortunately, while this may work in the short term, it means that we have not made any behavioural changes that will help us to keep the weight off in the long term.

For many of us having reached middle-age, we now have the freedom and finances to be able to go out socially. We consume more alcohol, take more holidays and cruises and generally indulge ourselves with the justification that we have worked hard and deserve it. Learning to make a few lifestyle changes allows us to enjoy our social life without gaining weight. Book me a table and I will meet you there.

Here are a few guidelines for dining out.

Visiting friends

Usually the dinner friends serve is simply that – a dinner. It is the nibbles that are eaten before the meal that are the problem. It would be easy to eat 1000 calories of chips and dips before dinner. So wait and eat the main meal.

When going out to dinner and not knowing what time we will actually eat, I find it useful to have a snack before I go out. I expand my late afternoon snack by adding grilled tomatoes to my toast or having a bowl of vegetable soup. It works like a little mini-meal. Thinking you will save up the calories of the day to blow at the dinner will mean that you sit down to the meal STARVING. Not a good strategy to start the night off.

Don't be coerced into having seconds – compliment your hostess on the meal and say it was so delicious you couldn't possibly fit in another mouthful. When praised, they usually leave you alone.

Restaurants

This is much easier because here we do have some control over what we eat. Unless you have been bound and gagged at the table, you are usually the person who orders the meal. Take responsibility for that.

Avoid starters like garlic and pizza bread. I would never eat bread before a meal at home so why fill up on it in a restaurant.

Try ordering two starters rather than a starter and a main.

If the dessert is to die for – have it. That is normal behaviour. It's no good being a goody-two-shoes at the restaurant and then going home and eating the whole two-litre block of ice-cream – in the dark. I am speaking from experience here!

Smorgasbord meals

Be selective. They don't put the soups, rolls and starters out to give you an extra treat. They are there to fill you so that you don't eat so much of the more expensive items. It becomes a game of beat-the-buffet. You have paid $25 for the meal and you want $45 value. The restaurant only want you to eat $15. You can't eat the entire buffet so go for the good stuff. Begin by serving yourself a seafood entrée of oysters, prawns and mussels. Then go back and dish up a delicious main course. Walk around the servery first before you start piling a load of mixed meals on your plate.

I have watched people return from the buffet with a meal that looked like they were eating the leftovers from the kitchen. Layers of ham, sweet and sour, prawns, salad, roast vegetables and chips. You can always return to the buffet but at least begin by dishing yourself a dinner that looks like a meal.

As for the dessert – check out the whole table. Make your choice and, if you don't like it leave it, and try another one. You don't have to eat it because you have taken it.

Eating out does not have to be a trauma. There will be times when we will eat more than is allocated on the food plan, but with wise choices we can minimise the damage and have a lovely meal. Keep in mind that it isn't what we do on that one night out, but what we do for the other 20 meals during the week that does the damage.

If you have over-indulged the night before
DON'T TRY TO STARVE IT OFF THE NEXT DAY.
Just get up and get back on the plan.

Alcohol

If you know that you have a heavy social calendar coming up, save some of your alcohol allowance for those nights. At least that will mean you start off with four drinks and, yes, we know you will sometimes exceed that, but at least it is only a few over the top.

I was once asked if a glass of wine could be substituted for a piece of fruit. My answer was: 'If you can take 12 grapes and turn them into a glass of wine – go for it!'

However, for many of us a glass of wine at the end of a busy day is like a 'decompression' between home and work. It may also mean that we stop, unwind, sit down and discuss the day with our families or just enjoy a quiet moment. It also means that we can enjoy a glass of wine when we are out socially without feeling deprived or left out.

Over-consumption of alcohol is the problem, not the odd glass. The key word here is MODERATION, but when it comes to alcohol consumption that is sometimes the challenge. Great intentions, one sip and who cares!

Research has found that in middle-age a MODERATE consumption of alcohol protects against heart disease, diabetes and blood-clot induced strokes. So the toast 'To your good health' does appear to have some legitimate validity. That's the good news. However, other recent research suggests alcohol, for women, increases the risk of breast cancer. Also to be considered is the weakening of willpower and the disruption to blood sugar levels. I hate to say this, but most of the health benefits favour men, wouldn't you know it!

If you were asked what was more fattening – a piece of cake or a glass of wine, you would probably say the cake. However, there is a bit of a double edge to the calorie consumption of alcohol compared with the cake. Alcohol is metabolised by the liver and turned directly into energy, not fat, meaning it doesn't contribute directly to our middle-age spread. While this may appear extremely positive news, there is a down side. When alcohol is present in the system it becomes the body's top priority fuel. This may be due to its potential toxic reaction in the body. Alcohol suppresses our body's ability to burn fat. One study found just three ounces of alcohol reduced the body's burning ability by one third. What this means is that while the body is burning alcohol it isn't utilizing the fats and other fuels and these are then stored on the abdomen. Talk about beer bellies!

Time for a reality check. What is considered moderation? For women, one glass of wine per day. On the Middle-Age Spread Diet we have allocated the option of using four choices of alcohol. Why only four when one a day is considered moderate? There's an obvious answer but I feel compelled to say it – BECAUSE WE WANT TO REDUCE OUR MIDDLE-AGE SPREAD.

Alcohol does not satisfy hunger or provide nutrients. If we lived off the alcohol we would suffer from malnutrition. One other factor we need to be aware of is that alcohol has 7 calories per gram. Compare that with carbohydrate, which has 4.5 calories per gram.

Each glass of alcohol contributes 100 calories to our day. If you enjoy a glass of wine every evening you have to weigh that up against how much weight you expect to lose. A glass of wine every night may result in a weekly loss of 200 to 300 grams, whereas if you stay within the allocated weekly allowance of four glasses of wine you could expect to lose 400–500 grams. Not a huge difference but over time it would make a difference to your overall loss.

My personal belief is that in order to be successful in the long term you have to integrate the diet into your individual lifestyle. If this means a glass of wine a night – accept the smaller loss BUT LIVE YOUR LIFE.

I have seen women take all the alcohol out, be miserable, lose the weight, put all the alcohol back in and with it the weight. Losing the weight with your lifestyle relatively intact will give you confidence in your ability to keep the weight off.

The old 'Chateau Cardboard' wine has a lot to answer for. A large, open, tapped supply of wine in the fridge has driven many of us to over-indulge. Go for quality not quantity.

Cheers!

Chapter 5

Maintenance

Maintaining Change

I believe **that anyone can lose weight but I** know **that not everyone will keep it off.**

I worked hard to achieve my weight loss and I am prepared to put the same effort into maintaining that loss. I don't allow my weight to rise more than one kilo before I swing into action. All the clothes in my wardrobe fit. I am ready for any special occasions, a wedding, school reunion or overseas holiday. Many people say how lucky I am to be still at this weight. Luck has nothing to do with it. I have chosen to stay at this weight.

How many times in the past have you managed to bring your weight down only to see your body slowly return to the old weight? Why didn't the weight stay off?

Ask yourself this question.

Did you continue to eat sensibly once you lost the weight? Think about that. Perhaps you had a glass of wine every night quickly followed by a little nibbly thing to go with it. You started eating a sweet biscuit with your cup of coffee each day. One day you ran out of Trim milk, and, oh dear, you are still using full cream. You thought it would be a change to cook your fish in batter and deep fry it (just for the family) and now it is the standard Friday-night dinner. I am constantly amazed that once having achieved our goal weight we seem to feel that it is 'over' and we can now return to our old eating habits.

Maintaining our weight is about maintaining the changes we have made. Weight does not go back on without some substantial help from us. If you have lost 15 kilos I can assure you that you will not just wake up tomorrow morning to find it has come back home from flatting and brought the washing with it! No. We give it lots of assistance, the key to the door, the fare home, and we vacate living space for the return. And then we bleat on and on about how it could have happened.

So how do we maintain?

Maintenance is understanding the energy balance.

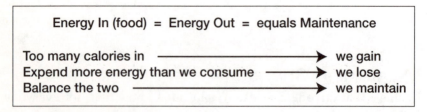

Understand this simple point and you have the secret of weight loss.

This energy balance will vary according to individual differences in the amount of exercise we are doing, our age and metabolic rate, and whether we are active in our jobs or sit at a desk.

▶ Maintenance is about learning what we can get away with, understanding our boundaries, and returning to within them after a holiday or night out. Be realistic about what you think you might be able to eat. We are not teenagers, and most of us are not running marathons or working in extremely physical jobs.

▶ Maintain with physical activity. Physical activity keeps the metabolic rate high and contributes to our maintenance. However, the emphasis must still be placed on the food intake with the exercise providing a helping hand in toning, shaping and fitness. I have visions of women pounding the streets so they can have more glasses of wine. They might end up with great legs but will still retain their middle-age spread.

▶ Maintaining does not require you to stay at home, locked in a room and being fed under the door!

▶ Maintaining does not mean deprivation – it means continuing to eat healthily with a few moments of madness thrown in.

Step up to maintenance

You have reached your desired goal weight and don't need to lose any more. It is now time to step up your daily food intake and to monitor the consequences.

If you achieved your weight loss following the

A List – you will step up to B List
B List – you will step up to C List
C List – you will step up to C Plus by adding in one extra food per day such as 1 Fruit or 1 bread or 1 glass of wine.

END-OF-WEEK EVALUATION

Weigh yourself at the end of one week.

A LIST
If your weight has gone **DOWN**	step up to List C
If you weight has gone **UP**	return to List A
If your weight has stayed the **SAME**	continue using List B

B LIST
If your weight has gone **DOWN**	step up to List C PLUS
If your weight has gone **UP**	return to List B
If you weight has stayed the **SAME**	continue using List C

C LIST
If your weight has gone **DOWN**	add in one more additional food each day.
If your weight has gone **UP**	return to List C
If weight has stayed the **SAME**	continue as the previous week

Continue to weigh and monitor the results at the end of each week. If you gain weight, take it off by dropping back to your original rating.

Be confident that your weight will not return, you have total control over the outcome, and a fast response to any gain will ensure your weight remains stable.

Get on the scales every week

Do not suffer from the Ostrich Syndrome – burying your head in the sand because it might be all too upsetting to see that the scales have gone up. You need to know they have gone up so that you can do something about it. Denial leads to massive weight gain and often our age gets the blame. Yes, our age does play a big part in the potential to gain, but only as a trigger to other factors, and we do have the ability to effect and maintain change.

Key points to remember

Weigh every week.

React quickly to any gains.

Add in additional foods slowly, monitor the outcome.

Continue with your physical activity levels.

Be confident of your success.

Chapter 6

Exercise

Exercise – it's a Breeze

Exercise, for our bodies, is like a breeze that fans the fire, ignites the energy and burns calories.

Think of a fire being piled up with fuel/energy (coal, wood) until it is choked and its ability to burn is stifled. It's very much like our bodies, overloaded, choked with fuel and with no breeze to fan the fire.

I have to admit that I have always been a reluctant exerciser. I have often found more good reasons for why I shouldn't drag my body out for a walk than good reasons why I should. It is easy to ignore the implications of this when we are young – but when middle-age arrives we wear the consequences. Gravity is a cruel master. The skin on our upper arms slides down to our elbows like an unwanted sleeve, our thighs sag towards the knees, we puff on the hills and we can no longer remove the lids from jars.

There is one over-riding reason why I made the decision to exercise. **Strength**.

And do you know that when I was young, the last thing I wanted to be was strong – strange how our priorities change. Now I am not talking about being built like a body builder – let's get real. It is more about maintaining and slightly building up the muscles that we already have. YES, there are muscles under that flabby skin, they are just shrivelling up from lack of use. It is estimated that between the ages of 35 and 80 we lose approximately 60% of our muscle strength.

One of the first indications, as we age, that we are losing strength in our bodies is our lack of balance. They say that once you have ridden a bike, you can always get on and ride again. Well – have you tried that recently? Riding a bike, skating, running, movement, all involve balance, and we find that as we age so do we fall.

Our balance, like our muscles, is in a constant state of decline, and we initially ignore the odd little trip or stumble. It is the first fall that brings it to our attention. It is the second or third fall that alarms us, and it is the fourth that puts us in plaster! Without reacting to these warnings, we compensate for our lack of balance by going slower, taking smaller steps, and going the long way around rather than taking the short cut. We develop a fear of falling and this can have a limiting effect on our wellbeing.

My motivation to exercise came directly from a series of falls. The first I dismissed as unlucky – I caught the heel of my sandal as I stepped over my herb garden and literally crashed down on my knees on a concrete path. Nasty! But then I shouldn't have been wearing heels in the garden!

The second fall was at the shopping mall – heels again, the patent leather caught on itself, and down I went.

Very embarrassing.

You know how you get up, dust yourself off and try to pretend nothing has happened. I threw the patent leather shoes away.

Third time lucky? Not quite. I was out walking when I came across a little stream. Walk around or jump it? Jump it! My right leg took the lead with my left leg crying out 'how does this go again?' The result was me face down in the stream. Mid-air indecision by a group of confused neurons and unco-ordinated muscles. My body was not balanced and it was definitely not strong enough to JUMP. Now I was a regular at the physiotherapist.

So let's recap. Why exercise?
▶ A strong body has better balance and a reduced risk of falling. Research findings report a 14% improvement in balance, muscle strength and alertness with regular exercise.
▶ Loss of muscle leads to fatigue.
▶ Exercises that strengthen our bodies increase our retention of bone density and help to minimise the risk of osteoporosis.
▶ Exercise improves lean body mass, which is metabolically active and burns more calories.
▶ Exercise moves the body as it is supposed to move and prevents us from seizing up.
▶ Exercise provides an outlet for built-up stress hormones.
▶ It develops a sense of wellbeing and encourages the release of our endorphins – our natural high hormones.

Research comparing the bone density of women who walked and those who didn't found that the walkers not only had strong leg bones but also strong forearm bones. This suggests that the message to retain calcium in the bones is not localised to the area of the body being worked but provides benefit to the whole body.

I want to debunk a few myths in relation to muscle and exercise.

Myth 1 – fat turns to muscle.
Wrong: We burn fat and we build muscle.

Myth 2 – weight loss after exercise is fat loss.
Wrong: Weight changes immediately after exercise do not reflect fat loss but rather dehydration. 1 kilo lost = 1 litre fluid loss

Myth 3 – age-related muscle loss cannot be regained.
Wrong: Weight-resistant exercise will develop and re-build muscles regardless of age.

How do we build muscles?

Muscles are bundles of fibres running in one particular direction.

Exercise triggers a message to the brain to lengthen or shorten a muscle to create movement. Muscle develops microscopic tears during movement. The body rebuilds and repairs the tear by producing new muscle fibres. The new repaired fibres are stronger and add to our muscle mass. It is due to the need to repair the muscle fibres that it is recommended that we leave a day in between our weight training to allow the body to recuperate.

Let's just go for a walk

Walking is becoming too technical for me – heart rate monitors, timing, pulse rates, did you drink your water, duration, frequency . . .

Rather than pounding the streets swinging our arms in some frantic fashion, why not just go for a walk. Is it such a radical thought? Whether you take a walk on your own or with a friend or family member, walking can be an energising and invigorating experience. It gives us a chance to escape the phone and leave the housework and our worries at home. We can familiarise ourselves with our neighbourhood, check out the neighbours' gardens and say hello to people in the street.

Choose the location for your walk based on your mood. On days that I need to scatter my cares in the wind, I drive to the local beach, take off my shoes and walk barefoot in the sand. It earths me. I take a brisk walk to the end of the beach, sit and contemplate on a rock, look at the birds and crashing waves, collect a couple of shells and then have a leisurely, relaxed walk back to the car.

You might find ways to incorporate exercise into your daily schedule.

At work – use stairs, park away from the office, indulge in window shopping and retail therapy around the shops in your lunch hour.

At home – cleaning, gardening, using the stairs, vacuuming, ironing – all these things use our muscles and increase our strength.

Weekends – enjoy a walk on the beach, a wander around streets and shops, play sport.

Don't underestimate the benefits of a regular walk. Studies have found that walking four times a week, for 45 minutes equates to an 8-kilo loss in a year. Your walks don't have to be tightly scheduled or monitored, but they should be regular. If you want to follow a more structured walking regime, I have placed a Walking Schedule on my website.

I met a woman recently who motivated me to continue walking. The first time I saw her she was walking briskly towards me and I had assumed by her posture and speed that she was a young woman. As we passed I was amazed to see that she was in fact quite elderly. Over several months we passed, occasionally nodded, but never spoke, until one day I discovered her resting at the end of the beach. It was an opportunity too great to miss, and, uninvited, I joined her. I said how impressed I was with her regular walks and speed and asked what motivated her.

'Simple,' she said. 'I set myself a little challenge that I refuse to let beat me. I have marked out my route and set a time on how long it will take me each day. I believe that if I walk every day there is no reason why I cannot continue to keep to that distance and time. I am seventy-three and age is not going to slow me down.'

Don't let age slow YOU down.

Walking has many benefits, but in order to build muscle we need to lift those weights.

Time to pump iron – and we aren't talking the steam iron!

Lower your weight by lifting weights.

We have stressed the value of exercise in raising the metabolic rate, maintaining lean body mass, de-stressing our bodies and raising our endorphins to feel good. Exercising with weights is now recognised as the most beneficial method for building muscles, and we have put together a simple set of exercises to help you tone and strengthen your body.

We recommend that you begin by exercising at least three times a week. Routine is everything. Set a specific time that you intend to exercise. Exercising in the morning invigorates you for the day ahead. However, if due to work commitments, this is not feasible, schedule a slot in the evening. Doing it regularly is more important than when you do it.

In the following exercises we have used two pieces of equipment that are readily available at good sports stores. Discuss your needs according to your level of fitness with a knowledgeable assistant. Do not buy weights that are too easy to lift because you will be surprised at how quickly your muscles grow stronger. You do not want to have to buy a heavier set too soon.

Weight bearing exercises increase bone density and have been found useful in preventing the onset of osteoporosis, which is a major problem affecting elderly people, mainly women.

Equipment to purchase:
- 2 dumb-bells
- 2 ankle weights.

You will also need:
- comfortable clothes and shoes
- a towel
- a sturdy chair for support.

We will start by performing two to three exercises every other day for the first two weeks. We will gradually increase the number performed until after six weeks you will repeat Days 35 and 37 on alternate days. See the Daily Exercise Schedule.

Daily Exercise Schedule

Don't forget to do the stretches before commencing each exercise.

Day 1	Biceps curls, Overhead triceps, Lunges
Day 3	Calf raises, Ballet dancer
Day 5	Inner-thigh firmer, Outer-thigh firmer
Day 7	Abdominal chair crunch, Waist side-swipes
Day 9	Repeat Day 1
Day 11	Repeat Day 3
Day 13	Repeat Day 5
Day 15	Repeat Day 7
Day 17	Repeat Day 1
Day 19	Calf raises, Ballet dancer, Inner-thigh firmer
Day 21	Outer-thigh firmer, Abdominal chair crunch, Waist side-swipes
Day 23	Repeat Day 1
Day 25	Repeat Day 19
Day 27	Repeat Day 21
Day 29	Repeat Day 1
Day 31	Repeat Day 19
Day 33	Repeat Day 21
Day 35	Biceps curls, Overhead triceps, Lunges, Calf raises
Day 37	Ballet dancer, Inner-thigh firmer, Outer-thigh firmer, Abdominal chair crunch, Waist side-swipes
Day 39	Repeat Day 35
Day 41	Repeat Day 37

Continue to repeat Days 35 and 37 on alternate exercise days.

Stretching

As we age our muscles become less flexible so it is important that we perform stretching exercises before working out.

We have given you the stretches that you require for each part of the body being exercised. There are only two exercises that do not require a specific stretch before beginning – these are the Biceps curls, the Outer-thigh firmer and the Waist side-swipe.

Do not hold your breath during stretch movements – breath normally.

Each stretch exercise must be performed twice before beginning and once again after you have finished the exercise.

Let us begin.

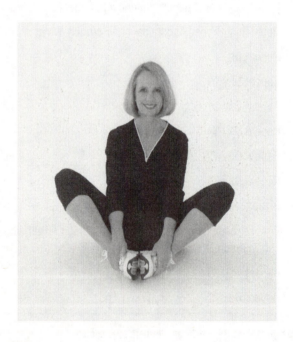

BICEPS CURLS

Tones: Front upper arm
Equipment: Two dumb-bells

▶ Stand with feet 20 cm apart.
▶ Begin by holding dumb-bells down each side of the body.
▶ Keeping upper arms close to the body, slowly raise right lower arm to chest level.
▶ Hold briefly and slowly return to starting position.
▶ Perform exercise 12 times. Repeat with left arm. Rest for 30 seconds.
▶ Repeat with each arm a further 12 times.

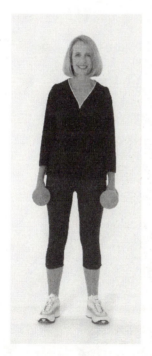 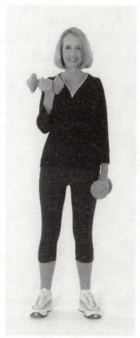

TRICEPS STRETCH

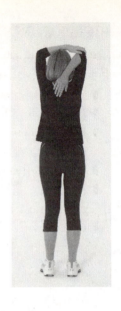

- Stand with feet together.
- Place right hand on back between shoulder blades.
- Grasp right elbow with left hand and gently push down on elbow until tension is felt in back of right arm.
- Hold for 30 seconds. Release. Repeat on left side.

OVERHEAD TRICEPS

Tones: Back upper arm
Equipment: One dumb-bell

- Stretch as above.
- Stand with feet 20 cm apart.
- Hold one dumb-bell in front of body with both hands.
- Keeping back straight and head facing forward, slowly raise arms to full length above head.
- Slowly lower dumb-bell towards back of neck.
- Hold briefly then slowly return to starting position.
- Perform exercise 6 times.
- Rest 30 seconds and repeat a further 6 times.

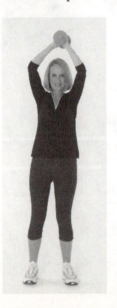
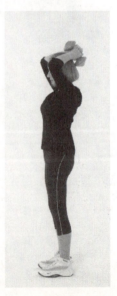

FRONT THIGH STRETCH

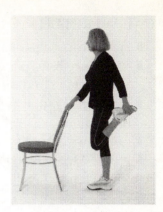

- Hold back of chair for support.
- Bend left knee so your left leg comes up behind you.
- Grasp left foot with left hand.
- Hold at point of tension for 30 seconds and release.
- Repeat with right leg and hand.

LUNGES

Tones: Front thigh
Equipment: Chair (optional – if you have difficulty balancing use the back of a chair for support.)

- Stretch as above.
- Place hands on waist.
- Keeping back straight, lunge right leg forward and drop left knee close to floor level with back foot heel raised off floor.
- Raise and lower left knee 6 times without changing the position of the right leg before returning to original position. Imagine a pulsing motion. The lower right leg must remain perpendicular and not lean too far forward. Make sure the leading knee does not extend past your toes.
- Repeat using the other leg.
- Rest 30 seconds.
- Repeat exercise with each leg.

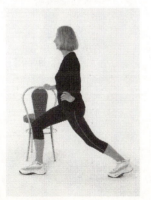
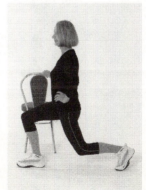

CALF STRETCH

- Hold back of chair for support.
- With knee bent, place right foot 30 cm in front of left leg.
- Hold left leg straight with foot flat on floor.
- Feel tension in calf of left leg.
- Hold 30 seconds and repeat with left foot.

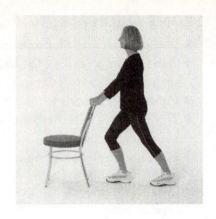

CALF RAISES

Tones: Calves
Equipment: Chair

- Stretch as above.
- Stand holding back of chair
- Rise onto toes, hold briefly and lower.
- Perform exercise 12 times.
- Rest 30 seconds
- Repeat a further 12 times.

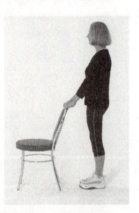 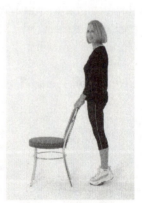

BUTT STRETCH

> ❱ Sit on floor.
> ❱ Cross right foot over left knee with left arm resting across outside of right knee.
> ❱ Without moving right knee, press left arm firmly against knee.
> ❱ Hold for 30 seconds. Release. Repeat using left foot.

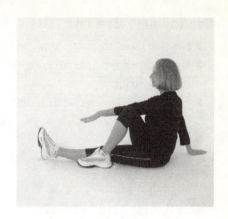

THE BALLET DANCER

Tones: Buttocks
Equipment: Ankle weights

> ❱ Stretch as above.
> ❱ Place ankle weight on each ankle.
> ❱ Place chair with back facing you.
> ❱ Stand with feet together 45 cm behind chair and hold back of chair with both hands for support.
> ❱ Keeping leg straight, raise left leg to back
> ❱ Squeeze your buttocks. Hold briefly.
> ❱ Return leg to starting position.
> ❱ Perform exercise 12 times.
> ❱ Repeat with right leg.
> ❱ Rest 30 seconds. Repeat a further 12 times with each leg.

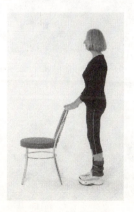 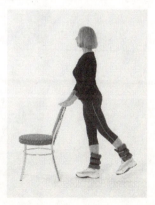

INNER THIGH STRETCH

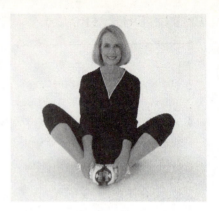

- Sit on floor.
- Knees bent to side with soles of feet together.
- Hold feet together with both hands for 30 seconds.
- Release.

INNER THIGH FIRMER

Tones: Inner thigh
Equipment: Ankle weights

- Stretch as above.
- Place ankle weight on each ankle.
- Lie on floor on left side with right leg bent so right foot is resting on floor behind left knee.
- Support head on left hand with left elbow resting on floor.
- Keeping leg straight, raise left foot 20 cm, hold briefly and lower to starting position.
- Perform exercise 6 times. Rest 30 seconds. Repeat a further 6 times.
- Repeat as above with right leg.

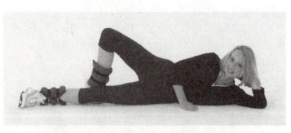

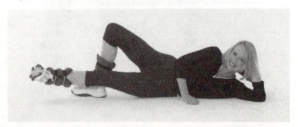

OUTER-THIGH FIRMER

Tones: Outer thigh
Equipment: Ankle weights

▶ Place ankle weight on each ankle.
▶ Lie on floor on left side.
▶ Support head with left hand and place right hand on floor at waist level.
▶ Bend left leg at right angle for support.
▶ Raise right leg as high as possible. Return to floor.
▶ Perform exercise 6 times. Rest 30 seconds. Repeat a further 6 times.
▶ Repeat as above with left leg.

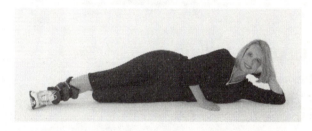

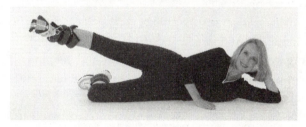

ABDOMINAL STRETCH

- ❱ Lie face down on floor.
- ❱ Lift and support upper body on forearms and elbows.
- ❱ BE CAREFUL NOT TO OVER-ARCH YOUR BACK.
- ❱ Keeping your abdominal area on floor and shoulders back, expand rib cage by taking a deep breath. Exhale.
- ❱ Hold position for 10 seconds continuing to breathe normally.

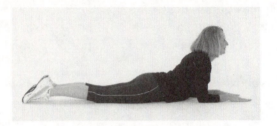

ABDOMINAL CHAIR CRUNCH

Tones: Firms and flattens stomach
Equipment: Chair

- ❱ Stretch as above.
- ❱ Lie on back on floor.
- ❱ Place lower legs on seat of chair.
- ❱ Place hands behind head.
- ❱ Holding lower back firmly against floor and keeping chin up, slowly raise the head and shoulders until you feel tension in stomach muscles.
- ❱ Hold for count of 2 and slowly return to starting position.
- ❱ Perform exercise 10 times. Rest 30 seconds. Repeat a further 10 times.

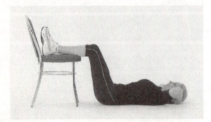 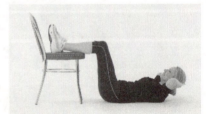

WAIST SIDE-SWIPES

Tones: Waist

- Stand with feet 30 cm apart.
- Place arms straight down against side of body.
- Slide right hand down body to thigh, as far as comfortable, hold briefly and return to start position. (Don't lean forward).
- Slide left hand down body to thigh, as far as comfortable, hold briefly and return to start position.
- Perform exercise 6 times. Rest 30 seconds. Repeat a further 6 times.

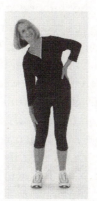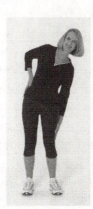

5 KEY POINTS TO REMEMBER

1. You are never too old to exercise. Exercise will increase your quality of life at any age.
2. Know you limits but don't underestimate your ability. If you tell yourself you can't do something you will not attempt it.
3. Don't give up. Think long term not just about the now.
4. Think of the benefits not the inconvenience. Nothing in life is easy but those who persevere succeed and reap the rewards.
5. As they say – it won't happen overnight but it will happen. Don't expect an overnight miracle; the 'muscle slip' didn't just happen and the reversal will take a little time also.

Exercises devised by Victoria Gibson-Clarke,
qualified fitness instructor and personal trainer

A wee story

I had an unfortunate experience the other day . . . It was at golf, it was a hot day and I had consumed quite a lot of water. There were people waiting on the tee behind us and my ball had gone down the hill. 'Run – hurry up,' my husband called, 'we're holding up the other players.' RUN! Off I went and as I did I had a 'wee' accident. Need I say more! Pelvic floor exercises suddenly took on new importance to me.

Exercise your pelvic floor

This routine is known as the Kegel exercise. It strengthens the pubococcygeus (PC) muscle, which is a layer of muscle that extends from the pubic bone in the front to the tailbone at the back.

This muscle layer forms the support structure for the bladder, bowel and uterus. When this muscle is strong it helps prevent bladder leakage and allows effective bowel and bladder emptying. Being overweight or physically unfit can contribute to pelvic muscle weakness.

First you need to identify the muscle we are talking about. You can do this quite simply next time you go to the bathroom. Start the flow of urine. Stop the flow, hold for 3 seconds, then restart the flow. The muscle you contracted is the PC muscle (Note: this is not the exercise). We are going to strengthen it through the following exercise.

1. Contract the PC muscle tightly and draw up internally.
2. Keep breathing and hold this contraction for the count of five.
3. Release hold and let muscle relax.
4. Rest for 10 seconds and repeat exercise.

As the muscle grows stronger hold for a longer period, up to 20 seconds, and repeat as many times as you feel able to, working up to 12 contractions. When you first begin, you may find it easier to perform this exercise sitting or lying down, but as your muscles grow stronger you can exercise standing up. It will take about three to six months to improve the muscle strength. Make a habit of always consciously tightening the pelvic muscle before you cough, sneeze, bend or do any heavy lifting.

This exercise can be done anywhere at anytime. The main thing is to do it every day for 5 to 10 minutes. You could exercise while watching TV – nobody will know.

Spring Cleaning
External housekeeping

There is a saying that states 'beauty is only skin deep'. As we age this saying has particular significance because our skin begins to lose depth and elasticity.

Some of the most attractive women are not what would be described as 'beautiful' and are definitely not young. They are, in fact, much more than that. They are healthy, vital, energetic, enthusiastic, toned and very much ALIVE. These women draw attention wherever they go – they are fun to be with and enjoy life.

What do they do? They take care of themselves, exercise regularly, eat healthily, remain interested in events around them and celebrate their age.

Taking care of our bodies is much more than going to the hairdresser or waxing our legs – much more and much more basic.

Cellulite — what is it?

Cellulite is a modified form of fat tissue that causes the skin to dimple and pucker. Located just below the surface of the skin, it is thought to be caused by poor circulation. It begins with the stagnation of blood in the capillaries and leads to a flow of blood fluids (plasma) through the capillary walls that separate our fat storing cells. Small groups of these cells become surrounded by micronodules, which are collagen fibre bundles. It is these bundles that cause the skin to be uneven and look like orange peel. As we age and our skin becomes thinner these bundles become more visible. Cellulite is a problem peculiar to women.

These fat cells and the connective tissue become the rubbish bin for our toxins, lymph fluid and cellular debris. Because these fat cells are metabolically less active than other cells in our body, they make an ideal location for the body's toxic waste, preventing it polluting the blood stream. This debris interferes with our DNA and results in early ageing.

Can it be fixed?

There is no quick remedy for removing cellulite as many people recently discovered when a highly publicised cellulite-removal drug was released on the market. I had women rushing up to me in the streets saying the miracle was coming as if it were a proven cure for cancer. People queued outside chemist shops to be first in just in case the shop sold out. The passing of time and consumer complaints have shown it to be totally ineffective.

A daily body rub is an effective means to improve our circulation and blood flow, and is reported to help eliminate cellulite. It also keeps our skin toned and minimises sagging and the formation of wrinkles.

Follow the procedure below for a few minutes each morning while in the bath or shower.

Use a loofah or body mitt, which you can buy at chemist or health stores. Do not rub where skin is broken or delicate.

1. Stand under warm shower so that your body is completely wet.
2. Rub some soap or shower gel on your mitt or loofah.
3. Begin at your shoulder and neck area. Using a circular movement, rub each shoulder several times. Move down each arm using long straight movements. Do not scrub one spot. Rub each elbow in a circular movement to remove any dead skin cells that build up here.
4. Gently rub across the chest.
5. Gently rub several times across the stomach and several times down. This movement helps with digestion and elimination.
6. Briskly rub the thighs and calves.
7. Rub the knees and ankles with circular movements.
8. Finish at your feet and rub both the upper and under part of each foot.

Internal housekeeping

Isn't it amazing how we talk about our bodily functions in hushed tones as if we were the only ones to experience them? Elimination of waste is one of those functions. We point to our distended abdomens and say 'look at my bloated stomach' when in fact the problem is more likely to be a clogged-up intestine.

When dealing with elimination problems, don't make excuses – lack of time being most popular. Make time. Schedule this important function into your daily routine. The elimination of waste matter from our system is vital to our good health.

I am going to be brutal here to hopefully jolt you into action. If you were given the option of carrying around a plastic bag filled with increasingly decaying waste OR taking five minutes each day to dispose of it, which would you choose? Don't let that waste linger in your body and become toxic to your system.

Constipation is a common complaint when diet or food intake is changed. This is especially true when there is a dramatic reduction in dietary fat.

Here are some guidelines to assist you.
If you experience ongoing elimination problems, it would be advisable to discuss them with your doctor.

Regularity	It is important to allocate a regular set time for elimination every day. To assist with regularity, select a time when you are not rushed or other people are waiting to use the bathroom.
	Eat 2 kiwifruit just before going to bed and 2 kiwifruit again first thing next morning – before eating or drinking anything else. If you find this over-compensates, then drop back to 2 kiwifruit either at night OR in the morning. Kiwifruit are very effective and are recommended to be eaten on a daily basis.
Exercise	A fit body will be more effective at elimination.
Diet	Eating a healthy, balanced diet containing fibre, fruits, vegetables and some fats will enable the body to function better.
Water	A consistent intake of water will keep the body hydrated and prevent dry stools leading to constipation.

As well as being important for internal housekeeping, water is vital for the overall good health of our body.

Water on the rocks

I have often said the best thing about drinking water is that it has no calories. These days, however, that statement could be challenged. If you are drinking the new sports waters or dietary supplements, then check the calories on the bottle – you may be surprised. One bottle I checked had 86 calories.

Sports drinks are useful if you are doing massive workouts and need fast replacement of fluids, but that probably doesn't apply to many of us. So don't let the benefits of no calories in the water be lost and think of all the money you will save.

If you live in an area where tap water is safe then my recommendation would be to use tap water in preference to commercial bottled water.

Unlike hunger, we cannot rely on thirst as a measure of our hydration level. Thirst occurs at 1% dehydration, and while this is not life threatening it can impede our performance and concentration. At a time when memory loss is already causing problems, it is worth ensuring the body is hydrated to avoid further impairment. I certainly need all the help I can get in the mental clarity area!

How much water should we be drinking?

Use common sense for your daily intake. If the weather is extremely hot, if you have been active, working out, sweating a lot, or been ill, then obviously you will need to replace those lost fluids. Even in winter months we can lose extra fluid, especially if we are working or living with central heating.

It is estimated that for each 250 calories we consume, we need approximately 1 cup of water. This means that if you were on a 2000-calories-a-day intake you would need 8 glasses. Very few of us are on 2000 calories a day, so it takes the pressure off this level of intake. Plus, on the diet plan, we are also consuming plenty of fresh vegetables and fruits, which have a high water content and boost our water intake.

Here is an estimate for you depending on whether you are A B or C.

A – drink 5 cups of water per day

B – drink 5 cups of water per day

C – drink 6 cups of water per day

Drink water for hydration and good health – not weight loss. One good reason to drink water is to prevent fluid retention. Seems a bit odd, doesn't it, to be told to drink more water when you are having difficulty getting rid of what you have. Cellular dehydration causes the release of an anti-diuretic hormone (AHA) from the posterior pituitary.

This causes the distal tubules of the kidney to be more permeable to water, which is then reabsorbed into the bloodstream resulting in concentrated urine and fluid retention. Natural diuretics include parsley, celery and watermelon.

How do you know if you are drinking enough? The colour of your urine should be consistently clear or a pale yellow. Remember though, that if you are using vitamin supplements they may cause your urine to be dark yellow or orange in colour, so take this into account.

Rethink how you are serving water.
Have you ever noticed how much water you get through if you are out at a restaurant and they place a bottle of iced water on the table? Often I prefer the water to the wine I'm drinking – so it has to be good! My favourite restaurant serves water in blue recycled wine bottles with a sea-shell collar and I have duplicated this at home. The blue bottle catches my eye in the fridge rack and reminds me to have another glass.

Try freezing a plastic bottle of water laced with lemon slices before you go to bed each night. In the morning, place it on the bench near the kettle so that as it thaws during the day you have cold, flavoured water easily accessible and acting as a memory trigger. Have a glass while waiting for the kettle to boil for your tea or coffee.

Freeze ice cubes with lemon slices, cucumber or strawberries to flavour your water and make it look more interesting.

If you are in a café or coffee shop ask for a glass of water with your espresso coffee. Coffee and tea act as diuretics and I always feel very 'dry' after I have drunk my short black. In Europe they nearly always serve water with coffee, a habit I never fully appreciated when I was there.

Heat it up. I didn't used to understand how anyone could drink plain hot water but I fully recommend it now. Small regular sips of very hot water every 30 minutes are suggested to be more hydrating and cleansing than drinking litres of cold water, and they help to flush out toxins and impurities in the system.

Try adding a slice of fresh root ginger to a cup of hot water – it's very refreshing, and ginger is excellent for our digestion and internal cleansing.

Chapter 7

Recipes

A Symphony of Grains, Seeds and Fruits

Cereal coated in honey, baked until caramelised, tossed with a few of my favourite things and served with a swirl of apricot yoghurt – who said they didn't like breakfast?

For 8 servings
1 cup rolled oats
2 cups Bran Flakes
4 teaspoons olive oil
3 tablespoons liquid honey
4 tablespoons raisins
6 dried figs, diced
12 apricot halves, sliced
2 tablespoons walnuts
1 tablespoon sunflower seeds
1 tablespoon pumpkin seeds

1. Pre-heat oven to 180°C.
2. In a large bowl combine the rolled oats and Bran Flakes.
3. In a cup mix together the oil and honey. Pour over the cereal mixture and toss to coat well.
4. Line an oven tray with baking paper and spread the cereal mixture evenly over the tray.
5. Bake for 5 minutes at 180°C, remove from oven and stir to turn cereal. Return to oven for a further 10 minutes. Stay with it and keep a close watch that it doesn't burn – it can turn from pale to burnt in the blink of an eye!
6. Remove from oven and allow to cool – stir to prevent cereal sticking together. Add the raisins, figs, apricots, walnuts, sunflower seeds and pumpkin seeds.
7. Store in an airtight container and enjoy eight days of delicious breakfasts.

Food allowance per serving
1 Breakfast Package = ½ cup cereal and ½ cup milk or ¼ cup yoghurt

Breakfast Pancakes with Lemon Honey

If you are home alone and want to make yourself a special breakfast, consider making this breakfast pancake stack and freezing the other three servings. It means you have three more breakfasts to look forward to without having to cook. There has to be something appealing about that.

For 4 servings – makes 8 pancakes
1 cup flour
2 teaspoons baking powder
pinch of salt
1 egg
4 teaspoons sugar
³/₄ cup milk (don't put it all in until you see how much you need)
2 teaspoons butter, melted (to put in pancake mixture)
2 teaspoons butter (to cook pancakes)

Lemon Honey
juice of 1 lemon
1 teaspoon lemon rind
4 teaspoons liquid honey
1 tablespoon water

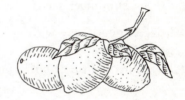

1. In a bowl sift flour, baking powder and salt.
2. In a bowl beat together the egg and sugar until thick.
3. Add egg mixture and milk to dry ingredients and mix until smooth. Stir in the first measure of butter.
4. Melt second measure of butter in non-stick pan and cook about one-eighth of mix on a medium heat. Turn when mixture bubbles burst. Repeat until all 8 are cooked.
5. In a small pot gently heat the lemon juice, rind, honey and water. Simmer on a low heat until syrup thickens. Serve poured over pancakes.

Food allowance per serving
1 Breakfast Package = 2 pancakes and lemon honey syrup

A Bit of a Mix-Up

This was one of those self-created recipes I invented when I wanted to get rid of three boxes of half-used cereal and felt they were greatly improved by being mixed together.

Mix together equal parts of the following cereals and store in an airtight container:
Ricies
Special K
San Bran

For one serving
½ cup A Bit of a Mix-up
2 dried apricots cut into small pieces
1 tablespoon raisins
1 teaspoon pumpkin seeds
1 teaspoon sesame seeds
1 teaspoon sunflower seeds

Mix together and serve with
¼ cup milk
2 tablespoons yoghurt swirled on top

Food allowance per serving
1 Breakfast Package

Bircher Muesli

This breakfast sticks to the sides and can be soaked the night before or made quickly and eaten in the morning. I'm not good at planning too far ahead so I make it in the morning.

For 1 serving
2 tablespoons rolled oats
1/4 cup milk
1/2 cup puffed wheat
1/4 cup fruit yoghurt
1/2 apple, grated
1/2 cup mixed berries – raspberries, boysenberries
1 teaspoon liquid honey

1. Place rolled oats in a serving bowl and pour the milk over. Leave to soak overnight or for at least one hour.
2. Fold in the puffed wheat, yoghurt and grated apple.
3. Top with berries and a swirl of liquid honey.

Food allowance per serving
1 Breakfast Package

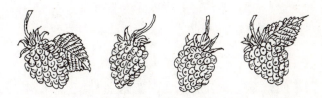

Gingered Fruit Compote for Breakfast

If you aren't a fruit person, but are craving something sweet, a fruit compote might just be the answer for you. This is a recipe I make in the winter and serve hot with a swirl of yoghurt on top.

For 1 serving
1 apple, peeled and sliced
2 figs, cut in halves
2 dried apricot halves
1 tablespoon raisins
1 teaspoon grated root ginger
1 teaspoon liquid honey
¹/₄ teaspoon cinnamon
¹/₄ cup natural yoghurt

1. Place the apple, figs, apricots, raisins, ginger, honey and cinnamon in a pot.
2. Pour in just enough water to cover and bring gently to the boil. Cover and simmer on a low heat for about 10 minutes. Keep a watch on the water level.
3. Serve hot or cold with yoghurt.

Food allowance per serving
1 Breakfast Package

Spiced Fillet-of-Beef Salad with Char-grilled Red Pepper Vinaigrette

For 4 servings

Spiced Fillet of Beef

2 teaspoons cumin
1 teaspoon coriander
3 cloves garlic, crushed
3 tablespoons lime juice
1 teaspoon crushed chilli
salt and ground black pepper
480 grams eye fillet (in the piece)

Char-grilled Red Pepper Vinaigrette

$1/2$ red pepper, deseeded, roasted, chopped
2 tablespoons olive oil
1 tablespoon white wine vinegar
1 tablespoon water
2 cloves garlic
1 teaspoon brown sugar
salt and ground black pepper

Salad

Lots of mixed greens – try mesclun salad leaves
$1/2$ red pepper, sliced
1 head broccoli, cut into small florets and blanched
$1/2$ bag aduki beans
handful of alfalfa bean sprouts

1. In a bowl mix together the cumin, coriander, garlic, lime juice, crushed chilli, salt and pepper. Rub onto the beef to coat well. Place beef on a plate, cover and refrigerate for a couple of hours.
2. Pre-heat oven to 220°C. Place beef in a roasting dish and cook for approximately 45 minutes or until cooked to your preference.

3. Use a blender to combine the roasted red pepper, olive oil, white wine vinegar, water, garlic, brown sugar, salt and pepper. Pour into a jar and place in refrigerator until ready for use.
4. While beef is cooking arrange salad ingredients on serving dish.
5. Thinly slice cooked beef and scatter over the salad.
6. Drizzle hot beef and salad with prepared dressing and serve.

Food allowance per serving
1 Protein = beef
1$\frac{1}{2}$ Fats = olive oil
$\frac{1}{8}$ Bit on the Side = brown sugar

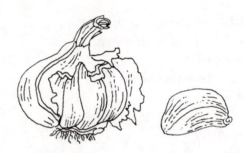

Tuscany Bolognaise with Farfalle Pasta $\boxed{\text{C}}$

This meal sounds pretty fancy for a spaghetti bolognaise but that's how exotic food is becoming these days. If you prefer you can use 480 grams beef mince rather than the beef and pork.

For 4 servings
4 teaspoons olive oil
240 grams beef mince
240 grams pork mince
1 red onion, finely diced
2 cloves garlic, crushed
2 x 400 gram cans tomatoes in juice
4 tablespoons tomato paste
1/2 cup red wine (optional)
salt and ground black pepper
120 grams Farfalle dried pasta (or spaghetti)
4 teaspoons grated Parmesan cheese

1. Heat oil in a non-stick pan and sauté mince, onion and garlic until lightly browned.
2. Add tomatoes and juice, tomato paste, wine, salt and pepper.
3. Cover and simmer gently for about 30 minutes – keep a watch on the fluid level so that it doesn't go dry. Top up with water if necessary. In Italy this sauce would simmer for 3 hours, but I can't wait that long!
4. While sauce is cooking prepare pasta following instructions on the pack.
5. Fold cooked pasta into the sauce and serve in large bowls sprinkled with the grated Parmesan cheese.

Food allowance per serving
1 Protein = mince (beef and pork)
1 Carbohydrate = pasta
1 Fat = oil
1 Bit on the Side = tomato paste and Parmesan cheese
1/4 Sheer Indulgence = wine (optional)

Corned-beef Hash Patties $\boxed{\text{C}}$

Cooking corned beef is so easy. Take a large pot of water, remove the corned beef from its plastic bag, drop it into the water with some peppercorns, an onion and some herbs and simmer gently for about 2 hours. I know it seems a long time but I am not suggesting you stand there and watch it. Go read a book. Serve hot corned beef one night and the next you can have leftovers, so two meals are solved in one hit. It leaves you time to read more of your book.

For 4 servings
300 grams corned beef, cooked and cut into small pieces
800 grams potato, peeled, parboiled and grated
2 eggs
1 onion, finely chopped
2 cloves garlic, crushed
2 tablespoons fresh chives, chopped
salt and ground black pepper
4 teaspoons flour, to dust patties
4 teaspoons butter, to cook patties

1. In a large bowl combine the corned beef, potato, eggs, onion, garlic, chives, salt and pepper.
2. Shape the mixture into 8 patties and lightly dust each with flour.
3. Melt butter in a non-stick pan and cook patties, turning only once, until golden brown on both sides.

Food allowance per serving
1 Protein = corned beef and eggs
2 Carbohydrates = potato
1 Fat = butter
½ Bit on the Side = flour

Smoked Chicken, Walnut and Potato Salad served tossed in Honey Mustard Dressing   C

Food should excite the taste-buds with its aroma, visual colour and texture. This recipe is the most amazing container lunch and can be easily prepared by cooking the potatoes the night before. You don't have to use smoked chicken – I usually make this from the left-over scraggy bits off my roast of chicken.

For 4 servings
400 grams smoked chicken, skinned and cut into chunks
880 grams gourmet potatoes, scrubbed, boiled in skins, halved
1 cup cherry tomatoes or 2 tomatoes cut into wedges
1 red onion, finely diced
2 tablespoons chives, chopped
3 tablespoons walnut halves, lightly chopped
big handful mesclun salad leaves

Honey Mustard Dressing
8 teaspoons olive oil
4 teaspoons wine vinegar
4 teaspoons water
2 teaspoons seed mustard
2 teaspoons liquid honey
salt and ground black pepper

1. On a large platter toss together the chicken, potatoes, tomatoes, onion, chives, walnuts and mesclun salad.
2. In a small jar combine the oil, vinegar, water, mustard, honey, salt and pepper.
3. Drizzle dressing over the chicken and potato salad – toss to coat well.

Food allowance per serving
1 Protein = chicken
2 Carbohdyrates = potato
2 Fats = oil
1 Bit on the Side = walnuts and honey

Arabian Nights Chicken Salad served on Lemony Fruit Couscous $\boxed{\text{C}}$

For 2 servings
240 grams chicken (about one double breast)
¹/₂ orange, juice and zest
¹/₄ teaspoon cinnamon
salt and ground black pepper

Fruit Couscous
³/₄ cup couscous (dry)
2 tablespoons raisins
2 dried figs, cut into quarters
2 tablespoons pine nuts
1 red pepper, cut in ¹/₂ and seeds removed
baby spinach leaves or mixed green salad leaves
handful parsley, finely chopped

Lemon Dressing
1 lemon, juiced
4 teaspoons olive oil
1 tablespoon water
pinch of salt and ground black pepper

1. Place chicken in a dish. Mix together the orange juice, zest, cinnamon, salt and pepper. Drizzle this over the chicken, cover and place in refrigerator to marinate for a couple of hours.
2. Pre-heat oven to 210°C. Place chicken in an ovenproof dish, cover and roast for about 45 minutes or until chicken is well cooked. About 15 minutes before the chicken is ready place seeded red pepper in oven to roast.
3. Prepare couscous following instructions on packet. Fluff it up with a fork as it absorbs the water. When water has been absorbed, fold in the raisins, figs, pine nuts, sliced roasted red pepper, spinach leaves and parsley.

4. To prepare the Lemon Dressing, combine the lemon juice, olive oil, water, salt and pepper in a small jar.

5. To serve: spoon couscous onto serving plate. Cut chicken into chunks and place on top of the couscous. Drizzle the Lemon Dressing over and lightly toss.

Food allowance per serving
1 Protein = chicken
2 Fats = olive oil
2 Carbohydrates = couscous
1¼ Fruits = orange and dried fruit
1 Bit on the Side = pine nuts

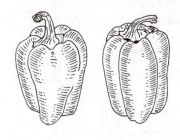

Chicken, Cashew and Pineapple Stir-fry

Change old habits – stir-fry meals don't have to be served with rice or a carbohydrate. Somehow I find the flavours and textures are accentuated when they aren't blended into the blandness of rice.

For 4 servings
4 teaspoons olive oil
480 grams chicken thigh or breast, cut into cubes
1 red pepper, sliced
1 green pepper, sliced
1 tablespoon grated root ginger
440 gram can pineapple pieces in juice (reserve juice)
2 tablespoons light soy sauce
2 teaspoons brown sugar
¹/₂ teaspoon crushed chilli
³/₄ cup water
2 teaspoons cornflour
1 teaspoon chicken stock
4 spring onions, diagonally sliced
2 tablespoons cashew nuts

1. Heat oil in a non-stick pan and sauté chicken until lightly browned.
2. Add green and red pepper and cook for a couple of minutes. Add grated root ginger and pineapple pieces and cook for a further 2 minutes.
3. Mix together reserved pineapple juice, soy sauce, brown sugar, crushed chilli, water, cornflour and stock. Pour into pan and stir until mixture comes to the boil.
4. Add the spring onions to the pan and simmer gently for 2 minutes.
5. Serve garnished with cashew nuts.

Food allowance per serving
1 Protein = chicken
1 Fat = olive oil
1 Fruit = pineapple pieces and juice
1 Bit on the Side = sugar, cornflour, cashew nuts

> On Carbohydrate nights you could add 1 cup cooked rice or 1 cup cooked pasta or 200 grams kumara cubes, steamed.

Chicken Thighs with a Coat of Many Spices

Years ago spices were something I bought to put in my fancy spice jars – all for show but I rarely used them. These days there is hardly a dish I don't throw a pinch of something into, transforming it into a divinely memorable meal.

For 2 servings
4 chicken thighs, skinned
2 teaspoons olive oil

Spicy Coating
1 teaspoon paprika
1 teaspoon ground ginger
1 teaspoon ground coriander
1 teaspoon ground cumin seeds
4 teaspoons flour
salt and ground black pepper

1. Pre-heat grill to 210°C.
2. In a shallow bowl mix the paprika, ginger, coriander, cumin, flour, salt and pepper.
3. Press the chicken thighs into the mixture and coat lightly but evenly.
4. Place chicken thighs on an oven tray, drizzle with oil and grill for about 8 minutes on each side or until the chicken is thoroughly cooked.

Food allowance per serving
1 Protein = chicken thighs
1 Fat = oil
1 Bit on the Side = flour

Chicken and Corn Pasta Salad   C

Go for double-up meals! They save time and solve the dilemma of what to have for dinner – twice. I cook a double portion of chicken so that I can serve a hot roast one night and then for lunch the next day I have cold chicken waiting for this salad. PLUS I can have it on the table in 20 minutes.

For 4 servings
400 grams cooked chicken, cut into cubes
3 cups penne pasta, cooked
¼ cup snowpeas – leave whole
1 red pepper, thinly sliced
1 cup baby cherry tomatoes or 2 tomatoes, cut in chunks
2 cups salad greens
1 cup sweetcorn, canned, drained

Yoghurt Dressing
1 cup natural yoghurt
4 teaspoons mayonnaise (try an interesting variety, such as Red Pepper)
juice and zest of ½ lemon
salt and ground black pepper

1. Toss together the chicken, penne pasta, snowpeas, red pepper, tomatoes, salad greens and sweetcorn.
2. To prepare the yoghurt dressing, mix together the yoghurt, mayonnaise, lemon juice and zest, salt and pepper. Fold through the salad and serve.

Food allowance per serving
1 Protein = chicken
2 Carbohydrates = pasta and sweetcorn
1 Fat = mayonnaise
1 Milk/Yoghurt = yoghurt

Gourmet Chicken Burger | C |

There is absolutely no competition between a homemade burger and a takeaway. Homemade wins every time and if you doubt that then you haven't tried this one.

For 4 burgers
360 grams chicken thighs
2 slices prosciutto or bacon
4 slices canned pineapple
4 hamburger buns
mesclun salad greens

Honey Mustard Sour Cream
4 tablespoons sour cream
1/4 cup natural yoghurt
4 teaspoons seed mustard
2 teaspoons liquid honey

1. Heat hot plate or grill and cook chicken until thoroughly cooked and juices run clear.
2. Cook prosciutto or bacon and pineapple on hot plate in the last 5 minutes of the chicken cooking.
3. Lightly toast hamburger bun. Top bottom half of bun with mesclun salad.
4. Place cooked chicken, prosciutto and pineapple ring on top.
5. Mix together the Honey Mustard Sour Cream ingredients and spoon over the top of the chicken.
6. Cover with the top half of the bun and serve.

Food allowance per serving
1 Protein = chicken and prosciutto/bacon
2 Carbohdyrates = hamburger bun
1 Fat = sour cream
1/4 Milk/Yoghurt = yoghurt
1/2 Fruit = pineapple ring
1/4 Bit on the Side = honey

Coconut Chicken with a Touch of Spice

For 4 servings
480 grams chicken thighs, cut into chunks
1 head broccoli, cut into florets and blanched
red pepper slices for garnish

Spice Marinade
¹/₂ cup natural yoghurt
1 red onion, finely chopped
1 teaspoon turmeric
1 teaspoon garam masala
1 tablespoon fresh coriander, chopped
1 teaspoon grated root ginger
2 cloves garlic, crushed
salt and ground black pepper
juice and zest of ¹/₂ a lime

Coconut Sauce
1¹/₂ cups Lite coconut milk
4 teaspoons peanut butter
1 teaspoon lemon grass, snipped (leave out if you don't have any)
2 teaspoons cornflour, mixed with a little water to form a paste
salt and ground black pepper

1. Place chicken in a large bowl.
2. In another bowl mix together the yoghurt, red onion, turmeric, garam masala, coriander, ginger, garlic, salt, pepper, lime juice and zest. Add to chicken and toss to coat well. Cover and place in fridge to marinate for several hours or overnight.
3. Pre-heat oven to 220°C.
4. Place chicken and marinade in an oven dish, cover and bake for about 30 minutes. Make sure it is well cooked.
5. In a pan heat the coconut milk and bring gently to the boil. Add the peanut butter, lemon grass, cornflour paste, salt and pepper. Cook on a low heat, stirring, until sauce thickens.

6. Add the chicken and broccoli to the pan. Simmer gently for about 5 minutes.
7. Serve garnished with slices of red pepper.

Food allowance per serving
1 Protein = chicken
1 Fat = peanut butter
2 Milk/Yoghurt = yoghurt and coconut milk
¼ Bit on Side = cornflour

On carbohydrate nights you could add 1 cup cooked rice or 100 grams noodles or 200 grams baked kumara or potato.

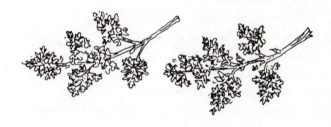

Chicken Waldorf Salad with Avocado and Lemon Dressing

It is said not to compare apples with pears, but when it comes to this recipe you can most definitely substitute one fruit for another. This combination of crisp gala apples and peaches is best when the produce is fresh, but don't let that slow you down as this recipe is delicious at any time of the year. Substitute melon or pawpaw for peach, and pears for apples if you wish.

For 4 servings
400 grams cooked chicken, cut into chunks
1 fresh peach, stone removed, cut into small chunks
2 gala apples, unpeeled, sliced thinly
12 green seedless grapes, whole
2 stalks celery, sliced in thin diagonal strips
3 tablespoons walnut halves, chopped
red coral lettuce or a fancy lettuce

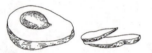

Avocado and Lemon Dressing

1 cup natural yoghurt   *¹/₂ teaspoon lemon zest*
3 tablespoons avocado   *1 tablespoon lemon juice*
1 teaspoon mayonnaise   *2 teaspoons liquid honey*

1. In a large bowl toss together the chicken, peach, apples, grapes, celery and ¹/₂ walnuts (hold some back for the top).
2. In a bowl combine the yoghurt, avocado and mayonnaise. Mash with a fork until smooth. Add the lemon zest, lemon juice and honey. Mix well.
3. Fold dressing through the chicken salad.
4. Arrange lettuce on a large serving dish and spoon chicken salad on top. Garnish with remaining walnut halves.

Food allowance per serving
1 Protein = chicken
1 Fat = avocado and mayonnaise
1 Fruit = apples, peach, grapes
1 Milk/Yoghurt = yoghurt
1 Bit on the Side = walnuts and honey

More Than a Roasted Chicken

A roasted chicken isn't very exciting, is it? In fact it is my default roast when lamb and pork are too expensive. This recipe gives roasted chicken new meaning.

For 4 servings
1 whole medium chicken
6 thin slices root ginger, cut into slivers
3 cloves garlic, cut into slivers
1 lemon
$1/2$ teaspoon paprika
$1/2$ cup natural yoghurt
2 teaspoons olive oil
$3/4$ teaspoon ground coriander
1 teaspoon cardamom
pinch of saffron threads (optional) or $1/4$ teaspoon turmeric
pinch of salt and ground black pepper

1. Pre-heat oven to 210°C.
2. Use a sharp knife to make small slits in chicken breast and insert slivers of ginger and garlic.
3. Place chicken in an ovenproof dish and squeeze lemon juice over. Tuck used lemon into the chicken cavity. Sprinkle chicken with paprika.
4. Mix the yoghurt, oil, coriander, cardamom, saffron, salt and pepper.
5. Spoon the yoghurt mixture over the chicken, cover, and bake at 210°C for $1^1/2$ hours.

Food allowance per serving
1 Protein = 100 grams chicken
$1/2$ Fat = oil
$1/2$ Milk/Yoghurt = yoghurt

Chunky Salmon Pâté $\boxed{\text{C}}$

If you are working and need a container lunch then this recipe is perfect. Select the carbohydrate of your choice from the following list. (They're in my order of preference.)

- ▶ 2 slices grainy bread, toasted
- ▶ 200 grams potato, baked crispy in jacket
- ▶ 20, yes, 20 small thin rice wafers
- ▶ 4 Ryvita crackers

For 2 servings
1 x 210 gram can salmon, drained
1 small onion, finely chopped
2 gherkins, finely chopped
1 tablespoon parsley, finely chopped
2 teaspoons cream cheese
2 tablespoons natural yoghurt
1 tablespoon lemon juice
1 teaspoon seed mustard
pinch of salt and ground black pepper

1. Place drained salmon into bowl and flake with fork. Remove skin and bones (my preference but leave bones if you like – they're a good source of calcium).
2. Fold in the onion, gherkins and parsley.
3. In a bowl combine cream cheese, yoghurt, lemon juice, mustard, salt and pepper.
4. Gently fold the dressing through the salmon mixture.
5. Refrigerate until ready for use.

Food allowance per serving
1 Protein = salmon
2 Carbohydrates = your choice from above
1 Fat = cream cheese
$1/4$ Milk/Yoghurt = yoghurt
$1/2$ Bit on the Side = gherkin

Baked Shrimp, Feta and Lime Parcels $\boxed{C}$

If you are not familiar with orzo, it is a pasta that looks like rice. It is found in supermarkets in the pasta section, and is usually in a box and sometimes called Risoni (which means, 'rice-like' in Italian). It's worth seeking out as it adds a new taste and texture to a meal.

For 2 servings
¹/₂ cup orzo pasta (uncooked)
2 teaspoons olive oil
2 tomatoes, finely chopped
4 spring onions, chopped
50 grams feta cheese, crumbled
juice and zest from 1 lime
salt and ground black pepper
120 grams shrimps, cooked
2 tablespoons basil, chopped
1 teaspoon olive oil (to drizzle over at the end)

1. Pre-heat oven to 210°C.
2. Cook orzo in boiling water for about 5 minutes. Drain and stir in 2 teaspoons olive oil.
3. Fold into the orzo the tomatoes, spring onions, feta cheese, lime juice, zest, salt, pepper, shrimps and basil.
4. Lay a long sheet of tinfoil in a baking dish. Line the tinfoil with a sheet of baking paper to prevent mixture from sticking.
5. Spoon the orzo and shrimp mixture onto the baking paper and fold up tinfoil to form a sealed parcel.
6. Bake at 210°C for about 25–30 minutes. Take care when opening the tinfoil to prevent a steam burn. Drizzle with the remaining teaspoon of olive oil and serve.

Food allowance per serving
1 Protein = shrimps and feta cheese
1 Carbohydrate = orzo pasta
1¹/₂ Fats = olive oil

Spiced Fish topped with Coconut Lime Raita

Put on those heels, get into the car and head to the shops to stock up on a few basic herbs and spices because we are going to create some exotic recipes. It is fun using spice, your food will smell wonderfully tempting and the taste is superb. Buy the spices!

For 4 servings
4 teaspoons butter
1 onion, finely chopped
3 cloves garlic, crushed
1 tablespoon root ginger, grated
360 grams fresh fish, cubed (try tarakihi or cod)
$^1/_2$ teaspoon turmeric
$^1/_2$ teaspoon cinnamon
$^1/_2$ teaspoon garam masala
$^1/_2$ teaspoon crushed chilli or powdered chilli
$^1/_4$ teaspoon ground cardamom
salt and ground black pepper
120 grams calamari rings
1 x 400 gram can savoury tomatoes
$^1/_4$ cup water
2 tablespoons tomato paste
1 tablespoon fresh coriander, chopped

Coconut Lime Raita
$^1/_4$ cup natural yoghurt
$^1/_4$ cup Lite coconut milk
juice and zest of 1 lime
2 teaspoons fresh coriander, chopped

1. Melt butter in a non-stick pan and sauté onion, garlic and ginger.
2. Add fish and sear for a couple of minutes to seal in juices.
3. Add turmeric, cinnamon, garam masala, chilli, cardamom, salt and pepper. Cook for 1 minute to develop flavours.
4. Add calamari and cook for a couple of minutes.
5. Add tomatoes, water and tomato paste. Simmer for 5 minutes than add coriander.

6. To make Coconut Lime Raita, in a bowl mix the yoghurt, coconut milk, lime juice, zest and coriander.
7. Drizzle Coconut Lime Raita over the fish and serve.

Food allowance per serving
1 Protein = fish and calamari
1 Fat = butter
$^1/_2$ Milk/Yoghurt = coconut milk and yoghurt
$^1/_4$ Bit on the Side = tomato paste

On Carbohydrate nights you could add 1 cup cooked rice or 1 cup cooked pasta or 200 grams baked potato.

Parmesan-crusted Pan-Fried Fish $\boxed{C}$

Of all the ways to cook fish I still prefer it coated in a crust and pan-fried. I could never eat fish steamed or poached – too white, too soft, not enough texture. Serve it with big wedges of lemon to squeeze over the fish and to bite into at the end.

For 2 servings
2 medium fish fillets approximately 280 grams (gurnard, snapper, tarakihi)
2 teaspoons flour
2 slices wholemeal bread, made into fresh breadcrumbs with a grater
2 teaspoons Parmesan cheese, grated
handful parsley, finely chopped
salt and ground black pepper
1 egg
¼ cup milk
2 teaspoons olive oil

1. Wash fish and pat dry on a paper towel.
2. Lightly dust fish with flour.
3. On a flat plate mix the breadcrumbs, Parmesan cheese, parsley, salt and ground black pepper.
4. Beat together the egg and milk.
5. Dip the fish into egg mixture.
6. Press the fish into crumbs on both sides to lightly coat.
7. Heat oil in a non-stick pan and cook for a couple of minutes on each side or until fish easily flakes and the crumbs are golden and crispy.

Food allowance per serving
1 Protein = fish
1 Carbohydrate = bread
1 Fat = oil
¼ Milk/Yoghurt = milk
1 Bit on Side = flour and Parmesan cheese
½ Sheer Indulgence = egg

Note: we have used one carbohydrate for the crumbs, which makes this meal a Carbohydrate meal. This does still leave you the option of using one more carbohydrate if you wish. You could serve one portion of potato, sweetcorn or kumara on the side or treat yourself to a dessert.

Smoked Salmon, Bacon and Dill Fettucine [C]

Mascarpone, if you haven't used it before, is a fresh, soft, creamy cheese that is unripened and melts down to form a sauce. It looks very similar to sour cream. I have allocated this as a protein rather than a fat.

For 4 servings
2 teaspoons olive oil
2 rashers lean bacon, chopped
50 grams mascarpone cheese
2 cups milk
4 teaspoons cornflour
salt and ground black pepper
240 grams smoked salmon, thinly sliced
2 fresh tomatoes, finely chopped
1 tablespoon fresh dill, chopped (or 1 teaspoon dried)
400 grams fresh fettucine
4 teaspoons grated Parmesan cheese

1. Heat oil in a non-stick pan and sauté bacon – don't allow to brown as this will discolour your creamy sauce.
2. In a bowl blend together the mascarpone cheese, milk, cornflour, salt and pepper. Pour into the pan and simmer on a gentle heat until sauce begins to thicken.
3. While sauce is cooking, prepare fettucine following instructions on the packet. Drain and keep warm.
4. Add smoked salmon, tomatoes and dill to the pan. Cook for a couple of minutes.
5. Fold cooked fettucine into the sauce and serve topped with grated Parmesan cheese.

Food allowance per serving
1 Protein = bacon, salmon, mascarpone cheese
2 Carbohydrates = fettucine pasta
$1/2$ Fat = olive oil
1 Milk/Yoghurt = milk
1 Bit on the Side = cornflour, Parmesan cheese

Chilli Prawn Pizza   C

Chilli is one of our metabolic boosters and when teamed with prawns and a mixture of cheeses it creates a delicious weekend lunch or casual dinner. If you don't have any mozzarella or brie you can use 200 grams of cheddar cheese.

For 4 servings
Pizza Base
2 cups flour
3/4 teaspoon baking soda
1 1/4 teaspoons cream of tartar
1 cup buttermilk OR 1 cup milk with 1 teaspoon vinegar

Base Spread
4 teaspoons basil pesto   *4 teaspoons cream cheese*

Chilli Prawn Topping
handful baby spinach leaves
1 red onion, finely sliced
120 grams chilli prawns, cooked
100 grams double cream brie, sliced
50 grams mozzarella cheese, grated

1. Pre-heat oven to 220°C.
2. To make pizza base, sift together in a bowl the flour, baking soda, and cream of tartar. Slowly fold in the buttermilk with a knife and mix to form a dough. Turn dough out on a lightly floured board and gently knead. Roll out into a large circle and place on an oven tray lined with baking paper.
3. Mix together the basil pesto and cream cheese. Spread evenly over base.
4. Cover the base with spinach leaves and top with red onion, prawns, brie and mozzarella.
5. Bake at 220°C for approximately 30 minutes.

Food allowance per serving
1 Protein = prawns, brie, mozzarella
2 Carbohydrates = flour
2 Fats = pesto and cream cheese
1/2 Milk/Yoghurt = buttermilk

Sesame Tuna Sushi   C

I have been a slow starter on eating sushi but I enjoy my own versions rather than the bought ones. This combination has a wonderful nutty aroma.

For 1 serving
1 cup cooked Calrose rice (can also use shortgrain or specialised sushi rice)
30 mls rice vinegar
salt to taste
1 sheet nori (dried seaweed)

Sesame Tuna Filling
1 tablespoon toasted sesame seeds
1 teaspoon tahini
50 grams tuna, drained
thin slices of red pepper, cucumber, spring onion

Dipping Sauce: (optional)
1/4 cup soy sauce, 1 teaspoon rice vinegar, 1/2 teaspoon grated root ginger, 1/2 red chilli, seeds removed and finely chopped, 1/2 spring onion, finely chopped

1. While rice is warm mix in the rice vinegar and salt to taste.
2. Place 1 sheet of nori on a bamboo rolling mat or a piece of baking paper.
3. Spread rice over two-thirds of nori sheet – taking it right to the outside edges.
4. On the halfway mark of the rice sprinkle the sesame seeds and drizzle a line of tahini. On top of this, place a line of flaked tuna and a layer of red pepper, cucumber and spring onion.
5. To roll up the sushi, firmly roll up from the edge nearest to you using your mat to keep the roll tight. Cut into 6 or 8 pieces.
6. Mix together the dipping sauce ingredients and serve in a small bowl on the side.

Food allowance per serving
1/2 Protein = portion of tuna
2 Carbohydrates = rice
1 Fat = tahini
1 Bit on the Side = sesame seeds

Fish and Chips for Dinner [C]

I have baked the fish in the oven so that I could use the oil for the chips.

For 4 servings
Seasoned Oven Fries
880 grams potatoes
4 teaspoons olive oil
1 teaspoon garlic salt
1 teaspoon sage
1 teaspoon thyme
pinch of cayenne pepper

1. Pre-heat oven to 220°C (on fan bake if you have it).
2. Peel potatoes, cut into thin wedges, and pat dry.
3. In a large bowl combine the oil, garlic salt, sage, thyme and cayenne pepper.
4. Add the potatoes to the bowl and, using your hands, toss the potatoes through the seasoning. Make sure all the potato wedges are well coated.
5. Spread wedges out on a baking tray and bake at 220°C for approximately 35–40 minutes or until crisp and golden. Give them a shake about half-way through the cooking to prevent them from sticking.

Herb and Lemon Fish Parcels
tin foil
480 grams (approx.) snapper fillets
4 tablespoons fresh oregano
2 onions, thinly sliced
juice and zest of 1 lemon
salt and ground black pepper

1. Cut 4 large squares of tin foil and place sliced onions in the middle of each sheet.
2. Lay a fillet of snapper on each square, sprinkle with oregano, a squeeze of lemon, zest, salt and ground black pepper.
3. Wrap tin foil to form a parcel and bake in oven with chips for 10–12 minutes.

Food allowance per serving of Fish and Fries
1 Protein = fish
2 Carbohydrates = potatoes
1 Fat = olive oil

Steamed Mussels with a Herbed Lemon Crust C

I enjoy eating mussels but until recently I was nervous about cooking them fresh in the shell and opted for buying them cooked and marinated – which isn't quite the same. Hand select your own mussels at the supermarket, making sure the shells are not cracked or broken – it's fun, gives you a sense of 'gathering your food' and they are in a taste league of their own.

For 1 serving
8 large mussels in the shell   *^{1}/$_2$ teaspoon peppercorns*
few sprigs of parsley

Herbed Lemon Crust
2 tablespoons fresh breadcrumbs
1 spring onion, finely chopped
1 clove garlic, crushed
juice and zest of 1 lemon
2 tablespoons coriander or parsley, finely chopped
1 teaspoon olive oil

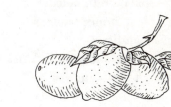

1. Pre-heat oven grill to 220°C.
2. Scrub mussels under running water and remove the 'beards'. Discard any mussels that have a broken shell or float rather than sink.
3. Place mussels in a large pan, cover with 1 cup of water, add peppercorns and parsley. Bring to the boil, cover with a tight fitting lid and steam for about 4 to 5 minutes. Give the pan a shake during this cooking time. Remove mussels from liquid and discard any that have not opened.
4. Use a sharp knife to remove the top shell. Lay the mussels on a grilling tray.
5. Mix together the breadcrumbs, spring onion, garlic, juice and zest, coriander and oil.
6. Sprinkle the mixture on top of each mussel.
7. Place under the grill and cook until the crumbs are crispy and golden.

Food allowance per serving
1 Protein = mussels
1 Carbohydrate = breadcrumbs
1 Fat = oil

French Lamb Cutlets with Herb Crust served with Creamy Minted Sauce

I rather fancy using French cutlets because they look attractive and don't have much fat on them to tempt me. However, when feeding the family the price can be prohibitive so you can use middle-loin chops instead.

For 2 serving
¹/₂ teaspoon dried mint
¹/₄ teaspoon turmeric
¹/₄ teaspoon chilli powder
1 teaspoon cumin powder
1 teaspoon flour
pinch of salt and ground black pepper
4 French lamb cutlets

Creamy Minted Sauce
¹/₄ cup natural yoghurt
2 tablespoons fresh mint, finely chopped
1 teaspoon vinegar
¹/₄ red onion, very finely chopped
¹/₂ teaspoon soft brown sugar

1. Pre-heat grill on high.
2. Mix together on a plate the mint, turmeric, chilli, cumin, flour, salt and pepper.
3. Press each cutlet into spice mixture to evenly coat both sides.
4. Place under grill and cook for approximately 5 minutes on each side or until cooked to your personal preference.
5. Combine all the sauce ingredients.
6. Serve the chops topped with mint sauce.

Food allowance per serving
1 Protein = lamb cutlets
¹/₂ Milk/Yoghurt = yoghurt
³/₈ Bit on the Side = flour and sugar

Marinated Teriyaki Lamb Stir-fry with Baby Beans

For 4 servings
480 grams lamb steaks, lean
2 teaspoons oil
2 bunches spinach leaves, washed and chopped
1 cup baby green beans

Marinade
2 tablespoons soy sauce
2 teaspoons olive oil
*2 tablespoons teriyaki sauce (available in sauce section at
    supermarket)*
juice of 1 lemon
1 tablespoon fresh mint leaves, chopped
2 cloves garlic, crushed
1 teaspoon ground cumin
pinch of cardamom

1. Trim any fat off lamb steaks and cut into cubes or thin strips.
2. In a bowl mix together the marinade ingredients. Add the lamb
   and toss to coat well. Cover and refrigerate until ready for use. Try
   to leave overnight if possible.
3. Heat oil in a non-stick pan. Drain meat and reserve marinade.
4. Stir-fry lamb until lightly browned and tender. Mix a little water
   with the marinade and add to the pan. Stir until sauce thickens.
5. Add spinach and beans to the pan and cook for 1 minute until
   spinach begins to wilt.

Food allowance per serving
1 Protein = lamb
1 Fat = oil
1/4 Bit on the Side = teriyaki sauce

On Carbohydrate nights you could add 1 cup Hokkien noodles or 1 cup
rice or 200 grams baked potato/kumara.

Grilled Lamb Burger with Mediterranean Vegetables

$\boxed{\text{C}}$

Save me from the washing up! This meal suits me – it's for one and is all cooked under the grill. There are no pots or pans to wash – just the grill. I make up the lamb patties in batches and freeze them for a quick no-mess meal. If you prefer you can use beef mince but lamb makes a nice change.

For 1 serving

Lamb Patty
120 grams lean lamb mince
1/2 small onion, peeled and chopped very fine
1 clove garlic, crushed
1 tablespoon parsley, chopped
1 tablespoon fresh mint, chopped
1/4 teaspoon ground allspice
salt and ground black pepper

Mediterranean Vegetables
1/2 red pepper, deseeded and cut in half
1 courgette, cut lengthwise into thin slices
1/2 small onion (other half used in burger), cut into slices
salt and ground black pepper

1 hamburger bun
1 tablespoon hummus

Mint Yoghurt Dressing
2 tablespoons natural yoghurt
few mint leaves, chopped
1 teaspoon lemon juice and 1/2 teaspoon lemon rind
pinch of salt

1. Pre-heat grill on high.
2. In a bowl mix together the lamb mince, onion, garlic, parsley, mint, allspice, salt and pepper. Shape into a hamburger patty.
3. Place patty under hot grill and cook for about 5 minutes.

4. Lay the pepper, courgette and onion on the grill beside the patty and sprinkle with salt and ground black pepper. Turn vegetables when you turn the patty.
5. Place hamburger bun under grill to lightly toast.
6. Prepare the mint yoghurt dressing by combining all the ingredients.
7. Spread hummus on hamburger bun. Place lamb patty on bottom half of bun, top with grilled vegetables and spoon the mint yoghurt dressing over the top.
8. Cover with remaining half of hamburger bun and serve.

Food allowance per serving
1 Protein = lamb
2 Carbohydrates = hamburger bun
1 Fat = hummus
$1/2$ Milk/Yoghurt = yoghurt

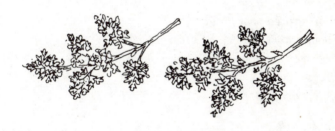

Marmalade and Ginger Pork Stir-fry

Marmalade is my favourite spread for toast and ginger is good for our digestion and health, so when teamed together in this stir-fry the result just has to be wonderful. You could use chicken if you prefer, but I find pork fillet tender, reasonably priced and a tasty alternative.

For 4 servings

Marinade

480 grams pork fillet, cut into chunks
$1/2$ teaspoon chilli powder
2 tablespoons soy sauce
pinch of salt and ground black pepper

4 teaspoons olive oil
3 cloves garlic, crushed
1 red pepper, thinly sliced

1 cup mushrooms, sliced
1 packet snowpeas
1 bunch spring onions, sliced

Marmalade and Ginger Sauce

1 tablespoon marmalade
2 teaspoons grated root ginger
3 tablespoons soy sauce
2 teaspoons soft brown sugar
1 cup water
3 teaspoons cornflour

1. Place pork in a bowl. Sprinkle it with chilli powder, soy sauce, salt and pepper. Cover and leave to marinate in the refrigerator for at least 30 minutes; overnight would be ideal.
2. Heat oil in a non-stick pan and sauté pork until cooked.
3. Add the garlic, red pepper, mushrooms, snowpeas and lastly the spring onions. Cook for a couple of minutes.
4. Mix together the marmalade, ginger, soy sauce, sugar, water and cornflour. Pour into the pan, and stir until sauce has thickened.

Food allowance per serving
1 Protein = pork
1 Fat = oil
1 Bit on the Side = marmalade, sugar and cornflour

On Carbohydrate nights you could add 1 cup cooked noodles or 1 cup cooked rice or 200 grams potato.

Glazed Marinated Pork Chop

I marinate my chop the night before so that the flavours have plenty of time to infuse into the meat. All I have to do when I get home is heat the grill, pop my chop under and then steam some vegetables while it's cooking – 15 minutes tops and I have a delicious meal on my plate.

For 1 serving
1 middle-loin pork chop, small

Marinade
1 teaspoon sesame oil
1 tablespoon soy sauce
1/4 teaspoon ground coriander
1/2 teaspoon soft brown sugar
pinch of Chinese five spice
1 clove garlic, crushed
pinch of salt and ground black pepper

1. In a bowl mix together the sesame oil, soy sauce, coriander, sugar, Chinese five spice, garlic, salt and pepper.
2. Press chop into the mixture to lightly coat each side. Cover and place in the fridge until ready for use.
3. Pre-heat grill on 220°C. Place chop on grilling tray and grill until well cooked on both sides.

Food allowance per serving
1 Protein = pork
1 Fat = sesame oil
1/4 Bit on the Side = sugar

Roasted Pork Fillet Mignon with Button Mushroom Sauce

Remember when we spent the whole day preparing for a dinner party? This is the perfect recipe for a stress-free dinner with friends and it always looks amazing.

For 4 servings
2 whole fillets of pork
6 sun-dried tomatoes, drained
4 tablespoons seed mustard
salt and ground black pepper
2 strips of bacon

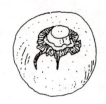

1. Pre-heat oven to 210°C.
2. Trim pork fillet and remove any fat or sinew.
3. Place a line of sun-dried tomatoes on pork fillet. Lay second pork fillet on top and press together.
4. Spread seed mustard over the outside of the fillet.
5. Wrap strips of bacon around fillet and secure with toothpick.
6. Cover and bake at 210°C for 30–45 minutes or until pork is cooked.

Button Mushroom Sauce
Make the mushroom sauce about 15 minutes before pork is ready.
3 cups button mushrooms, washed and left whole
1 cup water
1 teaspoon chicken stock
salt and ground black pepper
2 teaspoons cornflour mixed with a little water
handful of parsley, finely chopped

1. Place mushrooms, water, stock, salt and pepper in pot and bring gently to the boil. Simmer for about 5 minutes.
2. Add cornflour paste and stir until sauce begins to thicken.
3. Stir in parsley and serve mushroom sauce poured over the sliced pork fillet.

Food allowance per serving
1 Protein = 100 grams cooked pork and bacon
1/4 Bit on the Side = cornflour

Sweetcorn Fritters served with Ginger and [C] Chilli Sauce

While a sandwich is a good stand-by during the week it is nice to take the opportunity to enjoy a hot, cooked lunch at weekends. But for me it has to be quick and easy.

For 2 servings
$^1/_2$ cup flour
1 teaspoon baking powder
2 rashers lean bacon, chopped
2 eggs
$^1/_4$ cup milk
$^1/_4$ cup fresh coriander, chopped
1 teaspoon fresh root ginger, grated
2 spring onions, chopped
1 cup canned sweetcorn, drained
pinch of salt and ground black pepper
2 teaspoons olive oil

1. In a bowl sift flour and baking powder.
2. Heat a non-stick pan and sauté chopped bacon.
3. Lightly beat eggs and add cooked bacon, milk, coriander, ginger, spring onions, sweetcorn, salt and pepper.
4. Stir corn mixture into dry ingredients and mix well.
5. Heat oil in pan and spoon in mixture to make small fritters. Cook for several minutes on each side until lightly browned.

Ginger and Chilli Sauce

$^1/_2$ cup natural yoghurt
1 tablespoon fresh coriander, chopped

1 tablespoon sweet chilli sauce
$^1/_2$ teaspoon grated root ginger

1. Combine the sauce ingredients and serve drizzled over the corn fritters.

Food allowance per serving
1 Protein = egg and bacon
2 Carbohydrates = flour and sweetcorn
1 Fat = oil
$1^1/_4$ Milk/Yoghurt = yoghurt

Verde Fettucine with Ham and Mascarpone Sauce C

Believe me when I tell you that this is a fast recipe. I serve it piled high in large, chunky white soup bowls rather than on a flat plate. I'm sure there is some etiquette for eating fettucine, but I find serving it in a bowl and stabbing it with the fork does the trick. I prefer to use spinach fettucine to add colour – hence my title 'verde'.

For 4 servings
1 teaspoon butter
1 onion, finely chopped
150 grams shaved ham, sliced
3 tablespoons sun-dried tomatoes in oil
1 cup frozen peas
125 grams mascarpone cheese
salt and ground black pepper
400 grams fresh spinach fettucine
handful fresh basil leaves

1. Heat butter in a non-stick pan and sauté onion until soft.
2. Add sliced ham, sun-dried tomatoes, peas, mascarpone, salt and pepper. Stir on a low heat until mascarpone has melted into a sauce.
3. Cook fettucine following instructions on packet. Drain well and add to the pan.
4. Fold mixture together to coat well. Serve garnished with basil leaves.

Food allowance per serving
1 Protein = ham and mascarpone
2 Carbohydrates = fettucine
1 Fat = butter, and oil in sun-dried tomatoes

Spinach, Bacon and Avocado Salad with Creamy Mustard Salad Dressing

When I make this recipe I am usually asked if you can use silverbeet instead of spinach. My answer is no, not when served in a salad. It is a different matter if you are cooking with silverbeet but I find the flavour too strong for a raw salad. I know it is tempting when you have silverbeet growing in the garden, however don't compromise the flavour – buy the spinach.

For 1 serving
1 small bunch spinach, washed and torn into small pieces
few leaves of fancy lettuce
2 rashers bacon, grilled and chopped
¹/₄ avocado, cut into small cubes
1 stick celery, cut into thin slices
handful alfalfa sprouts

Mustard Salad Dressing
¹/₄ cup natural yoghurt
1 teaspoon mayonnaise
1 tablespoon balsamic vinegar
1 teaspoon seed mustard
salt and ground black pepper

1. On a serving plate mix together spinach and lettuce leaves.
2. Sprinkle lettuce with chopped bacon, avocado cubes and celery slices.
3. In a small bowl combine the yoghurt, mayonnaise, vinegar, mustard, salt and pepper.
4. Spoon Mustard Salad Dressing over the salad.
5. Garnish with alfalfa sprouts and serve.

Food allowance per serving
1 Protein = bacon
1 Fat = mayonnaise
1 Milk/Yoghurt = yoghurt
1 Sheer Indulgence = avocado

Give-me-a-Manhattan Toasted Sandwich $\boxed{\text{C}}$

When is a toasted sandwich a REAL toasted sandwich? When the butter runs down your chin. I have used two teaspoons of butter per serving – get your napkin ready!

For 2 servings
4 teaspoons butter
4 slices wholegrain bread
1 chorizo sausage, thinly sliced (you could use a bierstick)
50 grams mozzarella cheese, sliced
25 grams blue vein cheese, crumbled
1 char-grilled pepper, sliced (try the bought ones in a jar)
sprigs of fresh oregano or 1 teaspoon dried

1. Pre-heat a non-stick pan.
2. Soften the butter and spread it lightly on one side of each slice of bread.
3. Lay two slices of bread butter-side down, and layer with sausage, mozzarella, blue vein cheese, char-grilled pepper and oregano.
4. Top each with remaining slice of bread – butter side up.
5. Place sandwiches in pan, turn down heat, and cook until golden. Turn only once.
6. Slice each sandwich in half diagonally and serve piping hot.

Food allowance per serving
1 Protein = chorizo sausage and cheeses
2 Carbohydrates = bread
2 Fats = butter

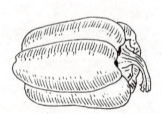

Greek Feta and Spinach Pie   C

Every time I make this pie I think of the movie *Shirley Valentine*. Did you see it? One Friday night she fed her neighbour's dog the steak she had bought for her husband's dinner. He was less than impressed by the eggs and chips she cooked him instead. Some family members (and I am not pointing the finger here) might not consider a dinner complete without a slab of steak on the side. Rather than never being able to enjoy this pie – slap a piece of steak or sausages under the grill and serve the pie to them as a side-dish.

For 4 servings
2 bunches spinach, washed and chopped
1 bunch spring onions, sliced
150 grams feta cheese, crumbled
2 eggs, lightly beaten
1 tablespoon fresh oregano chopped (or 1 teaspoon dried)
4 tablespoons sour cream
salt and ground black pepper
1/4 teaspoon nutmeg
4 tablespoons pine nuts, lightly toasted in a dry pan
8 sheets filo pastry
4 teaspoons butter

1. Pre-heat oven to 210°C.
2. Heat a little water in a non-stick pan and sauté spinach and spring onions until tender. Cook and press in a sieve.
3. In a large bowl combine the cooked spinach, onion, feta cheese, eggs, oregano, sour cream, salt, pepper, nutmeg and pine nuts.
4. Lay filo pastry on a flat board. Brush four sheets with melted butter and layer in an ovenproof dish.
5. Spoon spinach mixture into the pastry case. Brush the remaining four sheets with butter and layer on top of the spinach.
6. Bake at 210°C for about 30 minutes or until mixture is set.

Food allowance per serving
1 Protein = feta cheese and eggs
2 Carbohydrates = filo pastry
2 Fats = sour cream and butter
1 Bit on the Side = pine nuts

Gingered Buttercup and Cheese Fritters

I am an impatient cook and because of that I have had a few mishaps over the years. One was the result of my over-turning patties cooking in a pan. I have stressed this in the instructions below – turn them only once otherwise you will have to rename the recipe Buttercup Hash.

For 4 servings
400 grams buttercup
¹/₄ cup flour
¹/₂ teaspoon baking powder
salt and ground black pepper
3 spring onions, finely chopped
1 tablespoon sweet chilli sauce
3 teaspoons grated root ginger
150 grams tasty cheddar cheese, grated
2 eggs
8 teaspoons olive oil

1. Cut buttercup into large chunks and parboil until just tender. Allow to cool. Leave the skin on and grate back to the skin. (Leaving the skin on makes it easier to grate – discard the skin).
2. In a bowl sift flour, baking powder, salt and pepper.
3. Add the grated buttercup, spring onions, sweet chilli sauce, ginger and cheese to the flour mixture.
4. Separate eggs and mix yolk into the buttercup. Beat the egg whites until stiff and fold into the mixture.
5. Heat 4 teaspoons oil in non-stick pan. Place large spoonfuls of the mixture into the pan, flatten out slightly with the back of the spoon to form a fritter. Turn only once to prevent them breaking up.
6. Remove from pan and keep warm. When you have cooked half the mixture, add the remaining 4 teaspoons of oil to the pan and cook the remaining fritters.

Food allowance per serving
1 Protein = eggs and cheese
2 Fats = oil
1¹/₂ Bits on the Side = flour

Tomato, Basil and Ricotta Tart $\boxed{C}$

Tear some fresh basil leaves and smell the tantalising aroma of fresh herbs. After that you will never buy dried herbs again. My herb garden at home isn't very big (my friends call it a window-box), but it keeps me supplied with a mixture of fresh herbs all year. Keep planting every few months and try different varieties, such as red basil. Plant your own garlic cloves, lemon mint, garlic chives, Italian parsley . . .

For 4 servings
2 teaspoons tomato pesto
2 teaspoons olive oil
8 sheets filo pastry
1 small red onion, sliced and sautéed in a little water to soften
2 tablespoons fresh basil leaves – don't chop them, leave them whole
3 eggs
³/₄ cup milk
150 grams ricotta cheese
50 grams tasty cheddar cheese, grated
salt and ground black pepper
2 tomatoes, thinly sliced
2 tablespoons Parmesan cheese, freshly grated

1. Pre-heat oven to 210°C.
2. Mix together the tomato pesto and olive oil. Lay the filo pastry on a flat surface, brush each sheet with the pesto/oil mix and layer into an ovenproof dish.
3. Scatter the softened onions and basil leaves over the bottom of the tart.
4. Beat together the eggs and milk. Stir in the ricotta, cheddar cheese, salt and pepper. Pour mixture over the onions and basil and stir to combine.
5. Decorate the top with the sliced tomato and sprinkle with the grated Parmesan cheese.
6. Bake at 210°C for about 30 minutes or until mixture is set in the middle.

Food allowance per serving
1 Protein = ricotta, cheddar cheese and eggs
2 Carbohydrates = filo pastry
1 Fat = pesto and oil
³/₈ Milk = milk
³/₄ Bit on the Side = Parmesan cheese

Falafel with Minted Yoghurt Dressing

You have the choice with these falafel to either serve them as patties with salad and vegetables on the side or to tuck them in lightly toasted pita pockets. Some brands of chickpeas seem to be drier and have a tendency to crumble. If this does happen just spoon the 'crumble' into a pita pocket and drizzle with yoghurt – nobody will be the wiser.

For 2 servings
360 grams chickpeas, drained
3 spring onions, very finely chopped
2 cloves garlic, crushed
3 tablespoons parsley, finely chopped
1 tablespoon fresh coriander, chopped
$1/2$ teaspoon turmeric
2 teaspoons cumin
1 tablespoon sweet chilli sauce
1 teaspoon baking powder
pinch of salt
4 teaspoons olive oil

Minted Yoghurt Dressing
$1/2$ cup natural yoghurt
small handful fresh mint, chopped

1. In a blender process chickpeas to the consistency of breadcrumbs. Take care not to over-process as you don't want them ground into a paste.
2. In a bowl combine chickpeas, spring onions, garlic, parsley, coriander, turmeric, cumin, sweet chilli sauce, baking powder and salt.
3. Shape the mixture into 8 small patties.
4. Heat oil in a non-stick pan and cook the falafel on both sides until golden. Take care when turning the patties and try to only turn them once to prevent them breaking up.
5. In a small bowl combine the yoghurt and mint.

6. Serve falafel drizzled with the minted yoghurt dressing.

Food allowance per serving

1 Protein = chickpeas

2 Fats = olive oil

1 Milk/Yoghurt = yoghurt

On Carbohydrate nights you could add 2 small pita pockets or 1 medium pocket cut into 2 halves.

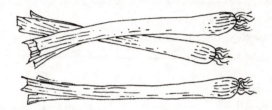

Lemony Orzo with Roast Pumpkin, Red Onion and Feta $\boxed{C}$

You could leave the orzo out if you wished to make this a Carbohydrate-free meal.

For 4 servings
1 large pumpkin wedge, peeled and cut into cubes
1 red onion, sliced
4 teaspoons olive oil
2 cups orzo pasta, uncooked
200 grams feta cheese, cut in small chunks
handful fresh mint, chopped
handful fresh parsley, chopped
4 tablespoons pine nuts

Lemony Vinaigrette
4 teaspoons olive oil
zest of ¹/₂ lemon
2 teaspoons cumin seeds
salt and ground black pepper

1 large lemon, squeezed
2 teaspoons water
2 garlic cloves, sliced

1. Pre-heat oven to 210°C.
2. Place pumpkin and onion in an ovenproof dish. Pour the oil over and toss to coat all the pieces.
3. Bake at 210°C for about 30 minutes or until vegetables have softened and lightly browned.
4. While vegetables are roasting, cook orzo following instructions on pack.
5. When vegetables are cooked place on a large serving platter and combine with orzo, feta cheese, mint, parsley and pine nuts.
6. Prepare the Lemony Vinaigrette: In a jar combine the oil, lemon juice and zest, water, cumin seeds, garlic, salt and pepper.
7. Pour dressing over the hot vegetable combination and gently toss to coat. Serve hot.

Food allowance per serving
1 Protein = feta cheese
2 Fats = olive oil
2 Carbohydrates = orzo pasta
1 Bit on the Side = pine nuts

Marinated Mushroom and Chickpea Salad

This is more my sort of food than my family's so I take the opportunity to enjoy it at lunch or for a Carbohydrate-free night. Chickpeas are an excellent source of isoflavones – it tastes wonderful and it's also good for you.

For 1 serving
180 grams canned chickpeas, drained
¹/₂ cup mushrooms, washed and quartered
¹/₄ cup parsley, chopped
1 teaspoon olive oil
1 tablespoon balsamic vinegar
1 teaspoon water
salt and ground black pepper
1 small red onion, quartered
2 tomatoes, cut into chunks
1 red pepper, cut into chunks
1 cup green beans, blanched
extra parsley
ground black pepper

1. Mix together the chickpeas, mushrooms and parsley.
2. Add the oil, vinegar, water, salt and pepper and fold into the chickpea mixture. Leave to marinate for about 30 minutes.
3. Place onion quarters under a hot grill to brown and soften.
4. On a serving dish layer the onion, chickpea mixture, tomatoes, red pepper and blanched beans.
5. Serve sprinkled with freshly chopped parsley and ground black pepper.

Food allowance per serving
1 Protein = chickpeas
1 Fat = oil

Grilled Caramelised Pear, Brie and Walnut Salad

Fruit, cheese and nuts make a delicious and simple combination. This is a dish I prepare for myself on weekends and serve with a chunk of freshly baked French stick.

For 1 serving
1 fresh ripe pear
1 tablespoon balsamic vinegar
1 teaspoon soft brown sugar
watercress or curly lettuce
50 grams brie or camembert cheese
1 tablespoon walnuts, roughly chopped
lemon juice (optional)

1. Pre-heat grill to 220°C.
2. Cut pear into quarters and remove the core.
3. Mix together the balsamic vinegar and brown sugar. Brush mixture onto cut surfaces of the pear.
4. Place pear on a grill tray and cook until caramelised and softened.
5. On a serving dish make a bed of the watercress or lettuce.
6. Arrange pear and brie on top and sprinkle with chopped walnuts.
7. Dress with a squeeze of lemon juice.

Food allowance per serving
1 Protein = cheese
1 Fruit = pear
1$\frac{1}{2}$ Bits on the Side = brown sugar and walnuts

A Many Bean Salad

We don't have to be a vegetarian to enjoy meatless meals, and for us, as middle-aged women, this is a healthy alternative. I am not into soaking and boiling the beans for hours so I simply buy a tin of mixed beans.

For 1 serving
180 grams mixed beans, drained
¹/₂ cup fresh/frozen whole baby green beans, cooked
2 tablespoons aduki beans
handful of mung bean sprouts
handful of alfalfa sprouts
¹/₄ red pepper, chopped
1 spring onion, chopped
1 tomato, diced
handful of parsley, chopped

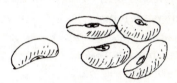

Balsamic Vinaigrette
1 teaspoon olive oil
1 teaspoon balsamic vinegar
1 teaspoon water
1 teaspoon seed mustard
1 clove garlic, minced
salt and ground black pepper

1. In a bowl mix together the chickpeas, green beans, aduki beans, mung beans, alfalfa, red pepper, spring onion, tomato and parsley.
2. In a jar combine the oil, balsamic vinegar, water, mustard, garlic, salt and pepper. Shake well and refrigerate until ready for use.
3. Toss dressing through salad just before serving.

Food allowance per serving
1 Protein = pulses (mixed beans)
1 Fat = oil

Crusted Tofu and Brazil Nuts with Stir-fry Vegetables

I know – tofu! And I am sure your initial reaction is 'no, thank you'. Tofu is an excellent source of phytoestrogens to boost our estrogen levels. I have found my enjoyment of eating tofu is based on how I slice it and cook it. Great chunks of white spongy tofu are definitely not for me – but crusted small cubes are totally different. One last thing – this is not a 'man's dish' and I haven't even considered serving it to my husband. It is my home-alone meal.

For 1 serving
120 grams tofu, cut into small cubes
1 teaspoon flour
1¹/₂ teaspoons sesame seeds
¹/₂ teaspoon paprika
1 teaspoon olive oil
¹/₂ teaspoon root ginger
¹/₄ broccoli head, cut into florets and blanched (to speed cooking)
¹/₄ red pepper, thinly sliced
¹/₄ cup snowpeas
1 spring onion, sliced
¹/₂ bok choy, sliced or spinach leaves
¹/₂ cup mung beans
3 brazil nuts, cut into halves
soy sauce (optional)

1. In a bowl mix together the flour, sesame seeds and paprika. Toss tofu in mixture to lightly coat.
2. Heat oil in a non-stick pan, add ginger and cook for 1 minute.
3. Add tofu and sauté until crisp and golden. Remove from pan.
4. Add broccoli and red pepper to pan and sauté for 2 to 3 minutes.
5. Add snowpeas, spring onion, bok choy and sauté for 1 minute.
6. Return tofu to pan and toss with vegetables to warm.
7. Add mung beans and brazil nuts to pan – toss until warmed. Serve with a dash of soy sauce if you wish.

Food allowance per serving
1 Protein = tofu and brazil nuts
1 Fat = oil
1 Bit on the Side = flour and sesame seeds

Herbed Soufflé Omelet with a Creamy Vegetable Salad Filling

This is one of my standby recipes for days when I want a light meal, don't feel like a sandwich, and most definitely don't want to spend time in the kitchen.

For 1 serving
2 eggs
2 tablespoons milk
2 tablespoons fresh herbs, finely chopped, e.g. oregano, chives, parsley
salt and ground black pepper

Vegetable Salad Filling
1 tomato, chopped in chunks
1/4 small cucumber, peeled and cut in small cubes
1 spring onion, finely chopped
4 mushrooms, sliced
2 tablespoons mixed bean sprouts
alfalfa sprouts
1 teaspoon basil pesto
4 tablespoons natural yoghurt
salt and ground black pepper

1. Separate eggs into two bowls. Beat the egg whites until stiff. Don't over-beat egg whites as they dry out and collapse. Beat the egg yolks with the milk. Add herbs, salt and pepper.
2. Gently fold the egg whites into the yolk mixture.
3. Heat a non-stick pan and pour in the omelet. Swirl pan to ensure an even spread of mixture. Tip pan to allow runny mixture to run underneath omelet.
4. Cook on a low heat for about 5–8 minutes or until the mixture is set.
5. While omelet is cooking, mix the tomatoes, cucumber, spring onion, mushrooms, mixed beans, alfalfa, pesto, yoghurt, salt and pepper.
6. Remove omelet onto a serving dish, spoon filling on one half and fold over.

Food allowance per serving
1 Protein = eggs
1 Fat = pesto
1/4 Milk/Yoghurt = milk

Hummus

I remember distinctly the first time I was served hummus, way back in the 1960s. I was taken to a Middle Eastern restaurant and there I was, all dressed up in my suit (short skirt – day of the mini), and I had to sit on a cushion! To cut a very long story short, when we were served the hummus with Lebanese bread, I couldn't believe anyone would ever be that hungry they would want to eat it. Now, not only have I discovered how delicious hummus is but also how good it is for us. Chickpeas are an excellent source of phytoestrogens, and tahini, which is sesame paste, is high in calcium. You can count one serving as a protein or 1 tablespoon as a fat.

For 2 servings
360 grams can chickpeas, drained (reserve some of the liquid)
2 cloves garlic, crushed
juice of 2 lemons
2 teaspoons tahini
1 teaspoon ground cumin
1 dash Tabasco sauce (optional)
¹/₂ teaspoon salt
reserved liquid from chickpeas

1. Place chickpeas, garlic, lemon juice, tahini, cumin, Tabasco sauce and salt in food processor. Blend until smooth.
2. Add enough of the reserved liquid from the chickpeas to make a creamy consistency.

Food allowance per serving
1 Protein = chickpeas
1 Fat = tahini

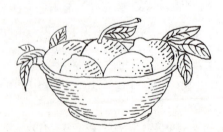

Spiced Lentil Soup with Crusty Garlic Butter Toast   C

A soup that combines all that is good for us makes the ideal lunch on a cold winter's day. Take it in a flask to work or heat it in the microwave – it's a complete meal combining protein, spices, carbohydrates and vitamins.

For 4 servings
2 teaspoons olive oil
1 large onion, finely chopped
1 clove garlic, crushed
1 teaspoon grated root ginger
1 teaspoon ground cumin
1/2 teaspoon cardamom
1 teaspoon turmeric
1 teaspoon mustard seeds
1 cup red lentils, washed
1 cup Basmati rice (well washed)
1 teaspoon vegetable stock
2 carrots, grated
4 stalks celery, finely chopped
2 cups baby spinach leaves
1 teaspoon salt
ground black pepper

Garlic Butter Toast
4 slices grainy wholemeal bread
2 teaspoons butter
2 cloves garlic, crushed
1 teaspoon finely chopped parsley

1. Heat oil in a large pot and cook onion, garlic and ginger until softened.
2. Add cumin, cardamom, turmeric and mustard seeds – cook for 1 minute.
3. Stir in red lentils, rice, stock, carrots and celery. Pour in just enough water to cover vegetables. Cover with lid and simmer gently for 30–40 minutes or until vegetables are soft. Use a potato

masher to blend into a chunky purée. I prefer the consistency to be chunky rather than using a processor and making it too smooth.

4. Add the spinach leaves and stir into hot soup – season to taste with the salt and pepper.
5. Serve with a slice of lemon on top.
6. **Garlic Butter Toast:** Toast bread. Use a fork to mash together the butter, garlic and parsley. Lightly spread garlic butter over the toast, cut into triangles and serve on the side of the soup.

Food allowance per serving
1 Protein = lentils
2 Carbohydrates = rice and bread
1 Fat = oil and butter

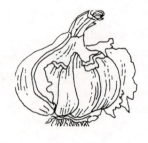

Chicken Laksa | C |

Most laksa recipes are made with seafood and fish sauce, which doesn't appeal to me in a soup. I much prefer this Chicken Laksa and it's a total meal – one pot and one bowl.

2 servings
2 teaspoons oil
220 grams chicken thighs, skinned and cut into cubes
2 cloves garlic
3 teaspoons medium curry powder
1 teaspoon curry paste
zest of 1 lime or ¹/₂ lemon, finely grated
1 tablespoon soy sauce
1 cup Lite coconut milk
2 cups water
1 teaspoon chicken stock
1 cup green beans
1 large carrot cut into sticks
salt and ground black pepper
200 grams Udon noodles
1 cup mung bean sprouts
handful of coriander leaves, chopped

1. Heat oil in a large pot and sauté chicken until lightly browned.
2. Add garlic, curry powder, curry paste and lemon zest. Cook for 1 minutes.
3. Add soy sauce, coconut milk, water, chicken stock. Bring to the boil.
4. Add the beans, carrot, salt and pepper. Cover and simmer for 40–45 minutes.
5. Add Udon noodles to pot and cook for a further 5 minutes.
6. Place ¹/₂ cup mung beans in each serving bowl and pour in hot soup.
7. Garnish with chopped coriander and serve.

Food allowance per serving
1 Protein = chicken
2 Carbohydrates = Udon noodles
1 Fat = oil
2 Milk/Yoghurt = Lite coconut milk

Pea and Ham Soup with Parsley Garlic Rolls   C

I like to make a big pot of soup and freeze a couple of servings for a fast lunch on a cold day. The fresh mint smells wonderful. Have you planted your herbs yet?

For 4 servings
1 large onion, chopped
2 carrots, grated
¹/₂ head of celery, chopped with green tops
1 cup yellow split peas
1 teaspoon chicken stock or vegetable stock
2 teaspoons grated root ginger
2 teaspoons ground cumin
2 teaspoons ground coriander
2 tablespoons fresh mint, chopped
salt and ground black pepper
water to cover
1 bacon hock

1. Place all soup ingredients in a large pot. Make sure the vegetables and hock are covered with water. Don't overfill with water as this will dilute the flavour of your soup.
2. Bring to the boil, cover and simmer for about 1¹/₂–2 hours. Keep a close watch on the water level and top up if necessary.
3. Remove bacon hock from the pot. Discard the skin and chop the bacon into small chunks.
4. Before returning bacon to the soup, lightly mash the vegetables to create a smooth consistency. Add the bacon and gently reheat for about 10 minutes.
5. Serve with the parsley garlic rolls on the side.

Parsley Garlic Rolls
4 wholemeal rolls
4 teaspoons butter
2 garlic cloves, crushed
chopped parsley

1. Pre-heat oven to 210°C.
2. Split roll in half.
3. Mash together the butter, garlic and parsley. Spread lightly on one half of each roll. Put two halves back together.
4. Wrap rolls in tin foil and bake at 210°C for about 10 minutes.

Food allowance per serving
1 Protein = split peas and bacon
2 Carbohydrates = roll
1 Fat = butter

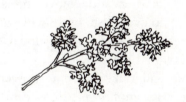

A Soup of Roasted Red Peppers and Tomatoes

When you serve this it may look like a tomato soup but the taste will be nothing like it. Gone is the acidity of the tomatoes and in its place a sweetness and a smooth velvety texture.

For 4 servings
4 red peppers
4 large tomatoes
2 teaspoons olive oil (1 tsp to brush vegetables and 1 tsp to sauté)
1 red onion, finely chopped
1 leek, white end only, chopped
1 clove garlic, crushed
1 teaspoon medium curry powder
¹/₂ teaspoon crushed chilli or ¹/₄ teaspoon chilli powder
2 tablespoons fresh basil
salt and ground black pepper

1. Pre-heat oven to 220°C.
2. Cut peppers into quarters and remove ends and seeds.
3. Place peppers in an oven dish, brush with oil and bake for 15–20 minutes. Brush the tomatoes with oil and add them half-way through the cooking time.
4. Remove peppers and tomatoes from the oven. Place peppers on a plate and cover with another plate to steam. This will help you to remove the skin. When peppers and tomatoes have cooled sufficiently to handle, remove the skins.
5. In a large pot heat remaining oil and sauté the onion, leek and garlic until tender.
6. Add the curry powder, chilli, basil, peppers, tomatoes, salt and pepper.
7. Pour in water to cover, and bring soup to the boil. Once soup is bubbling reduce heat and leave to simmer gently for about 20 minutes.
8. Remove pot from heat and allow to cool slightly. In a blender purée the soup in small batches until smooth. Return soup to pot and re-heat gently. Check seasoning and serve as an accompaniment to a meal.

Food allowance per serving
¹/₂ Fat = olive oil

Layered Hot Baked Potatoes for Lunch $\boxed{C}$

Cooking a baked potato for lunch is easier than it might seem. A quick zap in the microwave for about 8 minutes, slit it in two and drop your prepared filling on top.

For 1 serving
Bacon and Coleslaw Special
200 grams potato, scrubbed, pricked and baked in the microwave for about 8 minutes
2 rashers bacon, grilled and chopped

Coleslaw
1 cup cabbage, very finely sliced
1 tomato, cut into chunks
alfalfa sprouts
handful of parsley, chopped

1 carrot, grated
1 spring onion, chopped
small handful of aduki beans
1 tablespoon pumpkin seeds

1. Mix together all the coleslaw ingredients.
2. Split hot potato. Spoon coleslaw on top and sprinkle with crispy bacon
3. Spoon over Balsamic Dressing (refer page 203).

For 1 serving
Greek Combo
200 grams potato, prepared as above
125 grams cottage cheese or 50 grams feta cheese

Greek Salad
1 large tomato, cut into chunks
1 cup cucumber chunks
thin onion rings
4 black olives, cut into thin slices
handful of parsley, chopped

1. Mix together all the Greek Salad ingredients.
2. Split hot potato. Spoon Greek Salad on top.
3. Spoon cottage cheese on top and finish with Mustard Dressing (refer page 193).

Food allowance per serving
1 Protein = bacon OR cottage cheese
2 Carbohydrates = potato
1 Fat = olive oil in dressing
1 Bit on the Side = pumpkin seeds (coleslaw only)
= olives (Greek Salad only)

Roasted Spiced Potatoes   C

Crispy roasted potatoes are always delicious but if you are serving them with chicken or fish the coating of spices adds more flavour to the meal.

For 2 servings
2 teaspoons olive oil
1 teaspoon coriander
1 teaspoon cumin
¹/₂ teaspoon turmeric
¹/₂ teaspoon chilli powder
1 teaspoon mustard seeds (this is not the seed mustard but mustard seeds)
salt and ground black pepper
240 grams potato, peeled, dried and cut into quarters

1. Pre-heat oven to 220°C (fan-bake if you have it).
2. In a small bowl mix together the oil, coriander, cumin, turmeric, chilli, mustard seeds, salt and pepper.
3. Place potatoes in an ovenproof dish and brush with the spicy mixture.
4. Roast for 45 minutes turning from time to time to ensure even cooking.

Food allowance per serving
1 Carbohydrate = potato
1 Fat = oil

Potato Fritters with Lemon Sweet Chilli Sauce C

Cook these fritters slowly to ensure the potato is cooked in the middle of the fritter. You can parboil the potatoes first to speed things up if you wish but for me it's just another job.

For 1 serving
200 grams potato, peeled
1 courgette, grated
1 spring onion, chopped
2 eggs, beaten
2 tablespoons parsley, chopped
1 tablespoon flour
salt and ground black pepper
1 teaspoon oil

Lemon Sweet Chilli Sauce
juice and zest of half a lemon
1 teaspoon sweet chilli sauce
1/2 teaspoon soft brown sugar

1. Grate potatoes and squeeze out any excess moisture.
2. Place potatoes in a bowl with the grated courgette, spring onion, eggs, parsley, flour, salt and pepper.
3. Heat oil in a non-stick pan and spoon the mixture into four fritters. Flatten out with the back of a spoon. Cook on a moderate heat for about 5 minutes before carefully turning over. Cook for a further 6–8 minutes or until potato is cooked.
4. Mix together the lemon juice, zest, sweet chilli sauce and brown sugar and drizzle over the fritters.

Food allowance per serving
1 Protein = eggs
2 Carbohydrates = potatoes
1 Fat = oil
$1^3/_4$ Bits on the Side = sugar and flour

Vegetable Tabbouleh C

This recipe is one of my favourites and provides an excellent combination of phytoestrogens and colourful antioxidants. I always feel invigorated after eating tabbouleh and by making a double serving I have lunch ready for the next day. Add your own choice of protein to it – I usually add left-over chicken or feta cheese.

For 2 servings
1 cup burghul wheat
1 cup hot water with 1 teaspoon chicken stock
¹/₂ head broccoli, cut into small florets
1 courgette, cut into small chunks
¹/₂ cup chopped parsley
¹/₂ cup chopped coriander
¹/₄ cup chopped mint
2 spring onions, finely chopped
¹/₂ red pepper, seeded and diced
¹/₄ cucumber, peeled and cut into small chunks
1 medium tomato, cut into chunks
¹/₂ cup aduki bean sprouts

Dressing
2 teaspoons olive oil *2 teaspoons lemon juice*
zest of ¹/₂ lemon *2 teaspoons water*
1 clove garlic, crushed *salt and ground black pepper*

1. Place burghul wheat in a bowl and pour the hot water and stock over. Cover and leave to stand for about 15 minutes. Drain well and fluff up with a fork to separate the grains.
2. While the wheat is soaking, blanch the broccoli and courgette by dropping them in a pot of boiling water for about 2–3 minutes. Remove, drain and plunge them into a bowl of cold water to refresh and stop the cooking process.
3. Fold together the soaked burghul wheat, parsley, coriander, mint, spring onion, broccoli, courgette, red pepper, cucumber, tomato and aduki bean sprouts.
4. Mix together the oil, lemon juice and zest, water, garlic, salt and pepper. Pour dressing over tabbouleh and fold together.

Food allowance per serving
2 Carbohydrates = burghul wheat
1 Fat = oil

Vegetables Anyone?

If you have reached the point where you can't face another meal with carrots, peas and beans, then it's definitely time for a change. Like you, I needed a few quick combinations to break the daily monotony of steamed vegetables. Fill up your plate to the brim – all these recipes are created for ONE SERVING which you can multiply according to the number sitting down to dinner. All the recipes use 1 FAT from daily food allowance.

Roasted Vegetables (cook extra for a delicious sandwich, refer page 194)

1 teaspoon olive oil
1 courgette, cut into thin strips (try using a potato peeler to make ribbons)
1 carrot, cut into long thin strips
¹/₂ red pepper and ¹/₂ green pepper, cut into large chunks
1 small onion, peeled and cut into thick slices
I thin slice pumpkin/butternut, cut into strips
¹/₂ red chilli, seeds removed, finely chopped (optional)
salt and ground black pepper
handful of chopped parsley

1. Pre-heat oven to 210°C.
2. Lay vegetables in a roasting dish, brush with oil and sprinkle with salt and pepper.
3. Roast for 20 minutes, turning once to ensure vegetables are lightly browned.
4. Serve scattered with parsley.

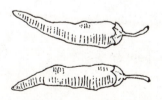

Smashed Carrots and Parsnip
2 carrots, scrubbed
1 parsnip, peeled
1 teaspoon butter
salt and ground black pepper
snipped chives or parsley

1. Cut carrots and parsnip into large chunks and cook in lightly salted water until soft.
2. Drain and mash with butter. Whip in chives and season with ground black pepper.

Bok Choy and Ginger
1 teaspoon olive oil
1 clove garlic, crushed
1 teaspoon grated root ginger
1 small head bok choy, trimmed and washed well, cut into chunks
pinch of salt and ground black pepper
soy sauce or oyster sauce

1. Heat oil in a non-stick pan and cook garlic and ginger for 1 minute.
2. Toss in bok choy and cook for 1 minute or until leaves wilt.
3. Season with salt, pepper and sauce of your choice.

Spiced Cabbage
1 teaspoon olive oil
1 small red onion, finely chopped
1 stick celery, finely chopped
1 teaspoon garam masala
$1/2$ teaspoon cumin
1 teaspoon sweet chilli sauce
wedge of cabbage, finely shredded
salt and ground black pepper
lemon juice

1. Heat oil in non-stick pan and cook onion and celery until soft.
2. Add garam masala, cumin and chilli sauce and cook for 1 minute.
3. Add shredded cabbage and cook for a couple of minutes until cabbage wilts.

4. Season with a pinch of salt, ground black pepper and a squeeze of lemon juice.

Red Pepper and Snowpeas
1 teaspoon olive oil
1 small onion, cut into thin slices
1 teaspoon grated root ginger
¹/₂ red pepper, cut into thin strips
¹/₂ green pepper, cut into thin strips
1 cup snowpeas, trimmed
pinch of salt and ground black pepper
soy sauce (optional)

1. Heat oil in a non-stick pan and sauté onion and ginger until tender.
2. Add sliced peppers and snowpeas and cook for about 2 minutes.
3. Season with salt and pepper and serve with a dash of soy sauce if you wish.

A Sauté of Tomatoes, Basil and Beans
1 teaspoon olive oil
1 small red onion, sliced
1 cup fresh or frozen green beans, steamed until just tender
2 tomatoes, remove skin and cut in chunks
salt and ground black pepper
basil leaves

1. Heat oil in non-stick pan and sauté onion until tender.
2. Add beans, tomatoes, salt and pepper and sauté for 5 minutes. Stir in basil leaves.

Roasted Beetroot
1 medium beetroot
1 teaspoon olive oil
salt and ground black pepper

1. Brush the beetroot with olive oil and sprinkle with salt and pepper.
2. Place in oven dish, cover with foil and bake at 220°C for 45 minutes.

Butter Up

Sometimes all a dish needs is a little buttering up. Create interesting toppings to spread on toasted French bread or to daub on top of vegetables, adding new flavours. Each of the following recipes is for FOUR servings. In each case, just mix all the ingredients together.

Char-grilled Red Pepper Butter

Try this butter spread on French bread and baked, or on top of a baked potato or with fish. For convenience I use bought char-grilled peppers bottled in oil, which I always have on hand in the refrigerator, or, if I am serving the dressing on page 159, I save a little of the peppers to use here.

4 teaspoons butter, softened
2 tablespoons roasted pepper, puréed
1 clove garlic, crushed
1 teaspoon parsley, very finely chopped

Cumin Butter

Let this butter melt into a hot corn-cob or crack open a hot jacket potato and drop a teaspoon on top.

4 teaspoons butter, softened
$1/4$ teaspoon cumin
2 teaspoons chopped coriander
pinch of salt and ground black pepper

Fiery Butter

This is my favourite on top of grilled fish.

4 teaspoons butter, softened
$1/4$ teaspoon harissa
1 clove garlic, crushed
squeeze lemon
$1/2$ teaspoon lemon zest

Food allowance per serving of butter
1 Fat = butter

Dressing Up

When you take the lid off these dressings you get the most wonderful whiff of garlic, mustard and herbs, which activates your taste-buds. It's a way to dress up a salad.

Vinaigrette/French Dressing

¹/₄ cup olive oil
¹/₄ cup balsamic vinegar
¹/₄ cup water
1 tablespoon seed mustard
2 cloves garlic, sliced
salt and ground black pepper

1. In a jar combine the olive oil, balsamic vinegar, water, seed mustard, garlic, salt and pepper. Shake well and store in refrigerator until ready for use.

Food allowance per serving
1 Fat = 4 teaspoons dressing

Classic Mayonnaise: 1 serving

¹/₄ cup natural yoghurt
1 teaspoon mayonnaise of your choice (try interesting blends, such as capsicum)
salt and ground black pepper

1. In a small bowl mix together the yoghurt, mayonnaise, salt and ground black pepper.

Food allowance per serving
1 Fat = mayonnaise
1 Milk/Yoghurt = yoghurt

Tangy Chilli and Lime Mayonnaise or Dip: 1 serving

¹/₄ cup natural yoghurt
1 teaspoon peanut butter
¹/₂ teaspoon sweet chilli sauce
zest and juice of ¹/₂ lime or lemon
1 teaspoon chives or parsley, finely chopped

1. In a small bowl mix together the yoghurt, peanut butter, sweet chilli sauce, lime zest and juice, and chives.

Food allowance per serving
1 Fat = peanut butter
1 Milk/Yoghurt = yoghurt

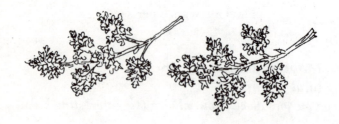

Grilled Sugared Cinnamon Peaches with Whipped Cream and Sliced Almonds

Grilling fruit intensifies the flavour and turns a fruit into a sensational dessert.

For 1 serving
1 fresh peach
1 teaspoon raw sugar
pinch of cinnamon
3 tablespoons whipped cream
¹/₂ tablespoon sliced almonds

1. Pre-heat grill on high.
2. Slice peach in half and carefully remove stone.
3. Mix together sugar and cinnamon (or use 1 tsp Vanilla Sugar, refer page 233).
4. Place peach halves in an ovenproof dish, sugared-side up. Grill on high until sugar has melted and peaches are lightly browned.
5. Spoon cream into each peach cavity and sprinkle with sliced almonds.

Food allowance per serving
1 Fruit = peach
1 Bit on the Side = sugar and sliced almonds
1 Sheer Indulgence = whipped cream

Cook's Note: Try this recipe with fruits in season – it's delicious made with bananas, nectarines or fresh apricots.

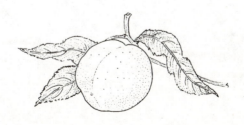

Roasted Macadamia and Fruit Cassatta

I first made this as a Christmas dessert but I enjoyed it so much I couldn't wait the 12 months to make it again. It is now one of my party pieces when I have friends over. When I want it to look special, I roll the mixture into balls, re-freeze them, then coat them in chopped nuts or toasted coconut. They look wonderful served in a tall parfait dish on a bed of fresh berries.

To make 2 litres
2 litres of French vanilla ice-cream
75 grams green glacé cherries
75 grams red glacé cherries
45 grams crystallized ginger
¹/₂ cup roasted macadamia nuts, roughly chopped
2 teaspoons ground ginger

1. Remove ice-cream from freezer and allow to soften for a couple of minutes. Spoon into a large bowl.
2. Into the ice-cream fold the green and red cherries, ginger, macadamia nuts and ground ginger.
3. Spoon the cassatta back into the ice-cream container and return to freezer until ready for use.

Food allowance per serving
1 Sheer Indulgence = ¹/₄ cup cassatta

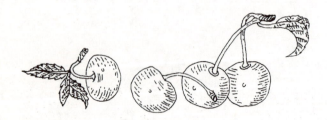

Mixed Berries and Apple Almond Crumble $\boxed{\text{C}}$

This recipe is one of my special treats at weekends and I like to make it in my two, small, deep, soufflé dishes as this way I get more crumble on top.

For 2 servings
1/2 cup stewed apple
3/4 cup mixed frozen berries
1 cup ready-made custard

Almond Crumble
1/4 cup flour
2 teaspoons butter
1 tablespoon demerara sugar (or soft brown sugar)
1 tablespoon sliced almonds

1. Pre-heat oven to 200°C.
2. In a small ovenproof dish mix the apple, berries and custard.
3. Rub butter into the flour, add sugar and almonds. Sprinkle crumble evenly over the fruit.
4. Bake at 200°C for about 20 minutes or until the fruit is hot and the crumble is lightly browned.

Food allowance per serving
1/2 Carbohydrate = flour
1 Fat = butter
2 Milk/Yoghurt = custard
1 Fruit = apple and berries
1 1/4 Bits on the Side = sugar and almonds

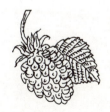 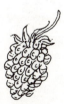 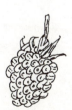 

A Touch of Wimbledon

Simple is so often best. When time runs out and you need a divine dessert, try fresh, seasonal fruit – strawberries are perfect – and dress in champagne.

For 1 individual serving
1 cup fresh strawberries
2 teaspoons Vanilla Sugar (refer page 233)
1 glass (104 mls) champagne or sparkling white wine

1. Wash strawberries, dry and remove hulls (hold back 1 whole strawberry).
2. Toss strawberries in Vanilla Sugar.
3. Pile strawberries high in a tall champagne flute.
4. Drizzle with chilled champagne or sparkling white wine.
5. Garnish with the remaining strawberry with its green top still on.

Food allowance per serving
1 Fruit = strawberries
1 Bit on the Side = sugar
1 Sheer Indulgence = sparkling wine

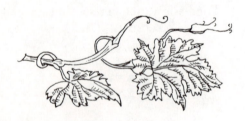

A Baked Apple Stuffed with Crystallized Ginger

For 1 serving
1 apple, preferably Granny Smith
1 tablespoon crystallized ginger, finely sliced
1 teaspoon liquid honey
pinch of cinnamon

1. Pre-heat oven to 180°C.
2. Remove the core from the apple. Slice off the bottom end of the core and insert back into the apple to form a plug.
3. Make an incision with the tip of a knife around the circumference of the apple.
4. Mix together the crystallized ginger, cinnamon and honey. Press into the centre of the apple. Cover opening with a little piece of foil.
5. Place apple in an ovenproof dish, add a little water and bake for 30–40 minutes until apple is soft and fluffy but not collapsed.

Food allowance per serving
1¹/₂ Fruits = apple and crystallized ginger
¹/₂ Bit on the Side = honey

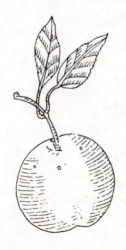

Ice-creams for Sheer Indulgence

I love ice-cream – too much at times. Have you ever served out the ice-cream for the family, measured out your portion exactly, then on the way back to the freezer quickly eaten a large scoop of the softened ice-cream from around the edge of the container? I have. By mixing up individual servings I can resist that feeling of 'just one last spoonful' and instead look forward to my own special treat.

Both these ice-cream mixes are for ONE serving.

Coffee and Walnut

¹/₄ cup vanilla ice-cream
1 tablespoon walnuts, chopped
¹/₂ teaspoon instant coffee dissolved in 1 teaspoon boiling water

1. Mix together all the ingredients, place in a covered container and keep in freezer until ready for use.

Food allowance per serving
1 Bit on the Side = walnuts
1 Sheer Indulgence = ice-cream

Sweet Summer Strawberries

¹/₄ cup vanilla ice-cream
1 cup strawberries
2 teaspoons caster sugar

1. Using a fork mash strawberries with caster sugar.
2. Fold the strawberries into the ice-cream, place in a covered container and keep in freezer until ready for use.

Food allowance per serving
1 Fruit = strawberries
1 Bit on the Side = sugar
1 Sheer Indulgence = ice-cream

Banana and Date Shortcakes $\boxed{\text{C}}$

Is it an afternoon tea or is it a dessert? BOTH. For a special treat, top with whipped cream or serve warm drizzled with yoghurt.

For 8 servings
2 cups flour
2 heaped teaspoons baking powder
pinch of salt
40 grams butter
2 tablespoons sugar
3/4–1 cup milk

Date and Banana Filling
2 cups dried dates
1/2 cup water
1 banana, peeled and mashed
1 tablespoon desiccated coconut

Cinnamon Sugar Topping (also delicious with Vanilla Sugar, refer page 233)
2 tablespoons raw sugar
1/2 teaspoon cinnamon

1. Pre-heat oven to 210°C.
2. In a bowl sift together the flour, baking powder and salt.
3. Rub butter into the dry ingredients. Add sugar.
4. Using a knife slowly cut the milk into the dry ingredients until mixture comes together. Add milk slowly as you may not need the full amount. You don't want the dough to be too wet or sticky.
5. On a lightly floured board gently knead dough to bring it together. Roll the dough out to a large rectangle shape.
6. To prepare the Date and Banana Filling, chop the dates and place in a pot with a little water. Simmer gently for about 5 minutes and mash with a fork to make them easier to spread. Allow to cool. Stir in the mashed banana and coconut.
7. Spoon the filling onto half of the dough. Gently fold the unfilled half over the date mixture to create a sandwich. Trim the edges.

8. Mix together the raw sugar and cinnamon and sprinkle over the top of the shortcake. You can either leave the shortcake whole or cut it into 8 servings.

9. Bake at 210°C for about 15–20 minutes or until golden.

Food allowance per serving
1 Carbohydrate = flour
1 Fat = butter
¼ Milk/Yoghurt = milk
1½ Fruits = dates and banana
1 Bit on the Side = sugar and coconut

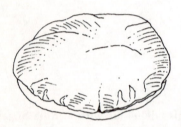
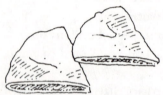

Blueberry Muffins C

When I am looking for variety in my fruit I often forget about berries – probably because they aren't available fresh all year. But they are a wonderful source of antioxidants, which are good for us so I have been buying them free-flow frozen. They don't go mushy, so I can use them in my fresh fruit salad or bake with them.

For 12 muffins (1 muffin = 1 serving)
2 cups flour
3 teaspoons baking powder
1 teaspoon cinnamon
1 cup Bran Flakes
4 tablespoons sugar
2 tablespoons butter
4 tablespoons liquid honey
³/₄ cup milk or buttermilk
1 egg
1 banana, mashed
³/₄ cup blueberries (frozen or fresh)

1. Pre-heat oven to 210°C.
2. In a bowl sift the flour, baking powder and cinnamon.
3. Add the Bran Flakes and sugar and stir to combine.
4. In a small pot melt together the butter and honey and add to dry ingredients.
5. In a bowl lightly beat together the milk and egg. Fold into dry ingredients.
6. Add the mashed banana and blueberries and fold gently to combine.
7. Spoon mixture into a lightly greased twelve-cup muffin tray.
8. Bake at 210°C for 12–15 minutes.

Food allowance per serving
1 Carbohydrate = flour and Bran Flakes
¹/₂ Fat = butter
¹/₆ Fruit = banana and blueberries
¹/₈ Milk/Yoghurt = milk
1 Bit on the Side = honey and sugar
¹/₁₂ Sheer Indulgence = egg

Ginger-beer Cake   C

I once ate a whole ginger-beer cake at the bus stop while waiting to go home with my shopping. I was young and foolish, say no more. But I still can see the look of horror on the faces of the people who were on the buses that went past me. It wasn't even that nice – but this recipe is. For ease of cutting I make it in my loaf tin, or if I need to take a plate I make mini-muffins, slice the tops and add a daub of cream. Sometimes I decorate them with a slice of ginger and serve them as fairy cakes.

For 8 servings
2 cups flour
2 teaspoons baking powder
1 cup ginger-beer
3 tablespoons sugar
2 tablespoons golden syrup
4 teaspoons butter
45 grams crystallized ginger, sliced
1 teaspoon baking soda
¹/₄ cup apple sauce (purée)
1 teaspoon icing sugar, to dust on top

1. Pre-heat oven to 180°C.
2. In a large bowl sift together the flour and baking powder.
3. In a pot heat together the ginger-beer, sugar, golden syrup, butter and crystallized ginger. When hot and melted, remove from heat and add baking soda.
4. Stir the cooled ginger-beer mixture into the sifted flour. Fold in the apple sauce and gently combine.
5. Line a loaf tin with baking paper. Spoon the ginger-beer cake evenly into the tin.
6. Bake at 180°C for 40–45 minutes. Check cake is cooked in middle before removing from oven.
7. When cake is cooled, dust top with icing sugar.

Food allowance per serving
1 Carbohydrate = flour
¹/₂ Fat = butter
¹/₂ Fruit = crystallized ginger and apple sauce
1 Bit on the Side = sugar, golden syrup and icing sugar
¹/₈ Sheer Indulgence = ginger-beer

Vanilla Sugar and a Few Little Sweet Things

Making Vanilla Sugar is so incredibly easy that I wonder why I took so long to do so. It's a wonderful treat in a jar waiting to be sprinkled on fresh fruits, breakfast porridge, cinnamon toast or enjoyed in a cup of coffee late at night. You can make it two ways – as I am doing by placing the pods in the sugar to infuse the flavour, or by popping the vanilla pods in a food processor until they're ground very fine, add them to the sugar and blitz again. I prefer it without the 'bits' in it, but it is more 'vanillary' when made that way.

To make 1 kilo
1 kilo caster sugar
2 vanilla pods

1. Fill an airtight jar with the sugar. Cut the pods in half and poke into the sugar.
2. Leave for about 2 weeks. It will keep indefinitely, and you can top it up from time to time.

Food allowance per serving
1 Bit on the Side = 2 teaspoons Vanilla Sugar

Cinnamon Toast for Afternoon Tea   C

For 1 serving
1 slice wholemeal bread, lightly toasted
1 teaspoon butter OR 1 teaspoon cream cheese
2 teaspoons Vanilla Sugar
½ teaspoon cinnamon

1. Lightly toast bread on both sides.
2. Spread with butter while still hot.
3. Mix together vanilla sugar and cinnamon and sprinkle over the toast.
4. Place under a hot grill for a couple of minutes to caramelise the sugar.

Food allowance per serving
1 Carbohydrate = bread
1 Fat = butter
1 Bit on the Side = sugar

Maple Fruit and Nut Loaf $\boxed{\text{C}}$

I have to say that baking is not my strong point. I would much rather cook a meal, but I always have success with a tea loaf recipe and my family enjoy having home baking in the tins.

For 8 servings
100 grams pitted dates, chopped
3 tablespoons soft brown sugar
1 tablespoon maple syrup (use golden if you don't have maple)
4 teaspoons butter
1¼ cups boiling water
1 teaspoon baking soda
2 cups flour
2 heaped teaspoons baking powder
½ teaspoon ground ginger
1 ripe banana, mashed
2 tablespoons walnuts, chopped

1. Pre-heat oven to 200°C.
2. In a bowl place dates, soft brown sugar, maple syrup, butter, boiling water and baking soda. Stir to combine and leave to cool.
3. In a bowl sift together the flour, baking powder and ginger.
4. When date mixture is cooled add to dry ingredients and mix well.
5. Lightly mash banana and mix together with the walnuts and fold into the mixture.
6. Lightly grease a loaf tin and spoon the mixture in evenly.
7. Bake at 200°C for 45–50 minutes – check with a skewer that it is cooked in the middle before removing from oven.

Food allowance per serving
1 Carbohydrate = flour
½ Fat = butter
1 Fruit = dates and banana
1 Bit on the Side = sugar, maple syrup and walnuts

Scones with Love and Lots of Kisses $\boxed{\text{C}}$

When I was cooking these scones on television, I had this brilliant idea of shaping the scones into hearts for Mother's Day. They looked wonderful going into the oven but I had not allowed for the fact that they would rise. They came out as irregular-shaped scones – not hearts. Go basic – cut them in squares.

Makes 8 scones
3 cups flour
1 level teaspoon baking soda
2 teaspoons cream of tartar
pinch of salt
40 grams butter
2 tablespoons sugar
1 egg
1 cup milk

Topping (optional)
8 teaspoons berry jam of
  your choice
8 tablespoons cream (plain
  whipped cream or clotted cream)
³/₄ cup berries

1. Pre-heat oven to 220°C.
2. Sift flour, baking soda, cream of tartar and salt into a large bowl.
3. Rub butter into dry ingredients until mixture resembles bread-crumbs. Add sugar.
4. Mix together the egg and milk and, using a knife, slowly add to the dry ingredients until mixture comes together. Note: you don't want the mixture too wet or the scones will be heavy.
5. Turn onto a lightly floured board and press out to form a rectangle.
6. Cut dough into 8 scones and place on an oven tray lined with baking paper.
7. Bake at 220°C in the middle of the oven for about 8–10 minutes or until lightly golden.
8. Allow scones to cool then cut in half. Spread each half with jam, cream and berries.

Food allowance per serving (1 scone)
1¹/₂ Carbohydrates = flour
1 Fat = butter
¹/₄ Milk/Yoghurt = milk
¹/₈ Fruit = berries
1 Bit on the Side = sugar and jam
¹/₂ Sheer Indulgence = egg and cream

Fruit Cake like Mother Used to Make   C

There is something about a fruit cake that makes me go a little crazy. Many moons ago when I was young and flatting in London, my mother sent me a cake for Christmas to share with my friends. It arrived on a day when I was at the flat alone and I ripped off the wrapping to be enveloped in the most wonderful smell of HOME. I will just have a little piece, I thought, before the girls get home from work. To prevent damage during shipping my Mum had baked it in the cake tin and I couldn't get the slice out. Then I heard my friends opening the front door. Like little Jack Horner, I grabbed a handful, stuffed it in my mouth, slammed the lid shut and kicked the tin under my bed. I never shared one crumb of that cake! Let me share this cake with you.

For 16 servings
1 kilo mixed fruit mix
2 cups orange juice
2 cups flour
2 teaspoons baking powder
1 teaspoon mixed spice
1/2 teaspoon cinnamon
1/4 teaspoon nutmeg
1/4 teaspoon almond essence
4 tablespoons soft brown sugar
glacé cherries for decoration

1. In a bowl combine the mixed fruit and orange juice. Cover and leave to soak overnight.
2. Pre-heat oven to 170°C.
3. Sift flour, baking powder, mixed spice, cinnamon and nutmeg into a large mixing bowl. Stir in almond essence, brown sugar and soaked mixed fruit.
4. Line an 8-inch square cake tin with baking paper. Spoon cake mixture evenly into tin. Decorate top of cake with glacé cherries.
5. Bake at 170°C for $1^1/4$ hours.

Food allowance per serving
1 Carbohydrate
1 Fruit
1 Bit on the Side
1/2 Sheer Indulgence

We are middle-aged, intelligent women, so let's act like it.

Cut a small slice, enjoy it with a cup of coffee, share it with friends and don't keep it under the bed.

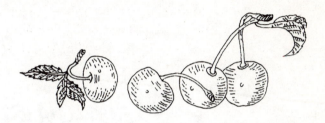

Conclusion

I changed my mind

I am a woman.

I am not only allowed to change my mind, but I am expected to, and when it comes to weight loss a change of mind is the secret of success.

Weight loss is achieved, not through the mouth,
but through our minds.

I asked you in my introduction to experience the difference between using the words 'I HAVE to lose weight' and 'I WANT to lose weight'. I hope you did this but, if you didn't, it's not too late to return to the introduction and do it now.

I believe in the basic philosophy that what you believe you can achieve, and if you can engender an emotional commitment and an attachment to that belief you will claim it as your own and succeed. I have proven this to myself on many occasions. Our minds contain years of expectations, disappointments and life experiences, which can, at times, cause us to question our ability to succeed. I know because I have also walked that path of self-doubt.

Losing weight is not about trying to reclaim our youth or become more attractive. What it is about is each of us being in control of our own body's requirements and making sure we provide ourselves with what we need for good health. It is said that we can neglect our bodies for our first 35 years and suffer the consequences for the rest of our lives.

Every week in my classes I meet women who arrive feeling bruised and disillusioned by their attempts to lose weight. Some of the methods they've used have been extreme and difficult to integrate into their lives. They failed.

I wrote the Middle-Age Spread Diet for myself – because I knew that if I could live with it, then so could you. We are not eating any diet products, artificial sweeteners, or low-fat foods. What we are doing is eating normally and in moderation.

I may at times, in an attempt to illustrate a point, appear to be light-hearted about weight loss. Scratch my surface and you will find I am intensely serious.

If you WANT TO LOSE WEIGHT then the path ahead is clear.

At the beginning I told you this book was about change.
I changed my mind and in turn it changed my life.

CHANGE.

For a change, why not come over to my place and visit me on the web?

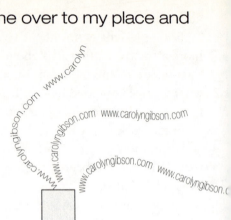

www.carolyngibson.com

I can help you with your equations, keep you stocked with planners and tempt your taste-buds with new recipe ideas.

Establish your:
▶ Waist to Hip Ratio (WHR)
▶ Body Mass Index (BMI)
▶ Calorie Expenditure
  Rating (CER)

Download:
▶ Personal Profile
▶ Analysis Sheet
▶ Food Planner
▶ Record Card

Plan your Exercise with:
▶ Walking Schedule
▶ Heart-rate Chart

Subscribe to FREE:
▶ Newsletters
▶ Recipes
▶ Updates
▶ Success Stories

Use my Conversion Calculator
Kilos/pounds/stone

Welcome

come on in

Appendix

Understanding our changes

Do you have a recurring symptom or behaviour – hot flushes, head-aches, sugar cravings, mood swings, depression? If so, write the symptom in the column headed Behaviour. Record the month and the date above the day you begin. Each day tick the relevant box depending on the symptom you are experiencing and monitor the pattern that emerges.

Being able to see a pattern of experienced symptoms could help you understand the underlying cause.

Although we stop menstruating we still retain a cycle. You may find, for example, that you experience severe sugar cravings every 21 days, and these may last for a week. Record this on your sheet.

I found this method of self-monitoring extremely helpful when I was experiencing continual migraines. I recorded a series of symptoms over a three-month time span. The outcome provided clear evidence the migraines were triggered by hormonal fluctuations and not food allergies or stress. This information is useful if you need to seek medical treatment. Understanding the pattern and possible causes allows us to be forewarned of potential risk times and to prepare ourselves to take preventative action.

Middle-Age Spread Personal Analysis Sheet

Behaviour	Mon	Tue	Wed	Thur	Fri	Sat	Sun	Mon	Tue	Wed	Thur	Fri	Sat	Sun	Mon	Tue	Wed	Thur	Fri	Sat	Sun
Month ( )																					
Month ( )																					
Month ( )																					

Selected Bibliography

Astrup, A. (1999). Physical activity and weight gain and fat distribution with menopause: current evidence and research issues. *Medicine & Science in Sports & Exercise*, Nov. 31, 11 Suppl: S564–67.

Beckham, N. (2002). *Menopause & Osteoporosis*. Victoria, Penguin.

Beckham, N. (1995). *Menopause*. Melbourne, Penguin.

Ben-Tovim, D. I., & Walker, M. K. (1994). The influences of age and weight on women's body attitudes as measured by the body attitudes questionnaire (BAQ). *Journal of Psychosomatic Research*, 38, 477–481.

Blaak, E. (2001). Gender differences in fat metabolism. *Current Opinion in Clinical Nutrition and Medicine*, 4, (6), 499–502.

Boellhoff-Giesen, C. (1989). Ageing and attractiveness: Marriage makes a difference. *International Journal Ageing and Human Development*, 29, (2), 83–94.

Brownell, K. D. (1991). Dieting and the search for the perfect body: Where physiology and culture collide. *Behaviour Therapy*, 22, 1–12.

Campbell, L. V., & I Samaras, K. (2000). What is the evidence, reasons for and impact of weight gain during menopause? *Medical Journal Australia*, Nov. 6, 173, Suppl: S100–101.

Chopra, D. (1994). *Perfect Weight*. London, Rider.

Chopra, D. (1993). *Ageless Body, Timeless Mind: A Practical Alternative to Growing Old*. London, Rider.

Coney, S. (1991) *The Menopause Industry*. Auckland, Penguin.

Connors, M. E., & Melcher, S. A. (1003). Ethical issues in the treatment of weight-dissatisfied clients. *Professional Psychology: Research and Practice*, 24, (4), 404–408.

Egger, G., & Binns, A. (2001). *The Experts' Weight Loss Guide*. Sydney, Allen & Unwin.

Egger, G., & Swinburn, B. (1996). *The Fat Loss Handbook: A Guide for Professionals*. Sydney, Allen & Unwin.

Fletcher, A. M. (1994). *Thin for Life*. Vermont, Chapters Publishing.

Garner, D. M., & Garfinkel, P. E. (1980). Cultural expectations of thinness in women. *Psychological Reports, 47*, 483–491.

Gibson, C. (1997). *The New Kiwi KISS Diet*. Auckland, Penguin.

Gibson, C. & Gibson, V. (1999). *The Kiwi KISS Workout*. Auckland, Penguin.

Heinberg, L. J., & Thompson, J. K. (1995). Body image and televised images of thinness and attractiveness: A controlled laboratory investigation. *Journal of Social and Clinical Psychology, 14*, (4), 325–338.

Herman, P., & Polivy, J. (1991). Fat is a psychological issue. *New Scientist*, Nov. 16, 35–39.

Hetherington, M. M., & Burnett, L. (1994). Ageing and the pursuit of slimness: Dietary restraint and weight satisfaction in elderly women. *British Journal of Clinical Psychology, 33*, 391–400.

Irving, L. M. (1990). Mirror images: Effects of the standard of beauty on the self and body-esteem of women exhibiting varying levels of bulimic symptoms. *Journal of Social and Clinical Psychology, 9*, (2), 230–242.

Ijuin, H., Douchi, T., Oki, T., Maruta, K., & Nagata, Y. (1999). The contribution of menopause to changes in body-fat distribution. *Journal Obstetrics & Gynaecological Research, 25*, (5), 367–372.

Kenton, L. (1996). *Passage of Power: Natural Menopause Revolution*. London, Vermillion.

Kimble, D. P. (1988). *Biological Psychology*. New York, Holt, Rinehart & Winston Inc.

Kirchengast, S., Grosschmidt, K., Huber, J., & Hauser, G. (1998). Body composition characteristics after menopause. *Collegium Anthropologicum*, Dec.; 22, (2), 393–402.

Ley, C. J., Lees, B., Stevenson, J. C. (1992). Sex and menopause associated changes in body fat distribution. *The American Journal of Clinical Nutrition*, May, 55 (5), 950–954.

Murillo-Uribe, A., Carranza-Lira, S., Martinez-Trejo, N., Gonzalez, J. (2000). Influences of weight and body fat distribution on bone density in post-menopausal women. *International Journal Fertility & Women's Medicine, 45*, (3), 225–231.

Nelson, M. E. (1997). *Strong Women Stay Young*. Melbourne, Lothian.

Ojeda, L. (1995). *Menopause Without Medicine*. Alameda, Hunter House.

O'Leary Cobb, J. (1989). *Understanding Menopause*. Toronto, Key Porter Books Ltd.

Plant, J. (2000). *Your Life in your Hands*. London, Virgin Publishing.

Rebuffe-Scrive, M., Lonnroth, P., Marin, P., Wesslau, C., Bjorn-Smith, U. (1987). Regional adipose tissue metabolism in men and post menopausal women. *International Journal of Obesity, 11*, (4), 347–355.

Rodin, J., Radke-Sharpe, N., Rebuffe-Scrive, M., & Greenwood M. (1990). Weight cycling and fat distribution. *International Journal of Obesity*, April; 14, (4), 303–310.

Sanson, G. (2001). *The Osteoporosis 'Epidemic': Well Women and the Marketing of Fear*. Auckland, Penguin.

Sanson, G. (1999). *Mid-Life Energy & Happiness*. Auckland, Penguin.

Schlosser, E. (2002). *Fast Food Nation*. London, Penguin.

Silverstein B., Perdue, L., Peterson, B., Vogel, L., & Fantini, D.A. (1986). Possible causes of the thin standard of bodily attractiveness for women. *International Journal of Eating Disorders, 5*, (5), 907–916.

Simkin-Silverman, L. R. & Wing, R. R. (2000). Weight gain during menopause: Is it inevitable or can it be prevented? *Postgraduate Medicine*, Sept; 1, 108, (3), 47–50, 53–56.

Toth, M. J., Tchernof, A., Sites, C. K., & Poehlman, E. T. (2000). Menopause-related changes in body fat distribution. *Annals of the New York Academy of Sciences*, May, 904, 502–506.

Toth, M. J., Tchernof, A., Sites, C. K., & Poehlman, E. T. (2000). Effects of menopausal status on body composition and abdominal fat distribution. *International Journal of Obesity, 24,* 226–231.

Tremollieres, F. A., & Pouilles, J. M., & Ribot, C. A. (1996). Relative influence of age and menopause on total and regional body composition changes in postmenopausal women. *American Journal of Obstetrics & Gynaecology,* Dec; 175, (6), 1594–1600.

Wang, Q., Hassager, C., Raven, P., Wang, S., & Christiansen, C. (1994). Total and regional body-composition changes in early postmenopausal women: Age-related or menopause related. *American Journal of Nutrition.* Dec; 60, (6), 843–848.

Waterhouse, D. (1998). *Outsmarting the Midlife Fat Cell.* New York, Hyperion.

Willett, W. C. (2001). *Eat, Drink and Be Healthy: The Harvard Medical School Guide to Healthy Eating.* New York, Fireside.

Zamboni, M., Armellini, F., Harris, T., Turcato, E., Micciolo, R., Andreis, I. A., & Bosello, O. (1997). Effects of age on body fat distribution and cardiovascular risk factors in women. *American Journal Clinical Nutrition,* July; 66, (1), 111–115.

Recommended Reading

Plant, J. (2000). *Your Life in Your Hands.* London, Virgin Publishing.

Sanson, G. (2001). *The Osteoporosis 'Epidemic': Well Women and the Marketing of Fear.* Auckland. Penguin.

Index

Recipe Index

Lamb

French lamb cutlets with herb crust served with creamy minted sauce	184
Grilled lamb burger with Mediterranean vegetables	186
Marinated teriyaki lamb stir-fry with baby beans	185

Mince

Grilled lamb burger with Mediterranean vegetables	186
Tuscany bolognaise with farfalle pasta	161

Pasta

Chicken and corn pasta salad	168
Chicken laksa	209
Lemony orzo with roast pumpkin, red onion and feta	200
Smoked salmon, bacon and dill fettucine	179
Tuscany bolognaise with farfalle pasta	161
Verde fettucine with a ham and mascarpone sauce	192

Pastry

Greek feta and spinach pie	195
Tomato and basil ricotta tart	197

Pizza

Pizza base	180
Chilli prawn pizza	180

Potatoes

Layered hot baked potatoes for lunch	213
– Bacon and coleslaw special	213
– Greek combo	213
Potato fritters with a lemon sweet chilli sauce	215
Roasted spiced potatoes	214
Seasoned oven fries	182

Pork

Glazed marinated pork chop	189
Marmalade and ginger stir-fry	188
Roasted pork fillet mignon with button mushroom sauce	190

Rice

Salads

Sauces

Soups

Stir-fries

Vegetarian

Vegetables

Kiwi KISS
ALL SEASONS
COOKBOOK
CAROLYN & VICTORIA GIBSON

Kiwi KISS is a proven diet and exercise programme used successfully by thousands of New Zealanders.

Follow the Kiwi KISS plan for health and fitness with a cookbook that celebrates the benefits of eating fresh, seasonal food. Whether you are savouring a luscious strawberry or enjoying the warmth and comfort of a delicious home-made soup, the *All Seasons Cookbook* encourages you to look forward to each changing season with a sense of anticipation and delight.

Carolyn Gibson is the creator of Kiwi KISS and the author of the best-selling *Kiwi KISS Diet Book*. Victoria Gibson writes and develops new recipes for the Kiwi KISS plan, is a qualified personal trainer and co-author of the *Kiwi KISS Workout Book*. Victoria achieved a weight loss of 28 kilos on the Kiwi KISS programme and has maintained this for 11 years.

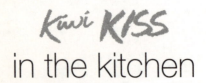

Kiwi KISS
in the kitchen
CAROLYN GIBSON

Designed to fit the KISS Diet plan, here are great tasting recipes for soups, appetisers, main meals, snacks, desserts and more that will be enjoyed by everyone, whether slimming or not.

And the Kiwi KISS Diet *does* work! Thousands of New Zealanders have achieved their slimming and lifestyle goals through following Carolyn Gibson's successful recipe of commonsense eating, good food and a dash of 'can do' attitude.